Pamela B. Carter

Editor

Guide to Physical Fitness and Exercise

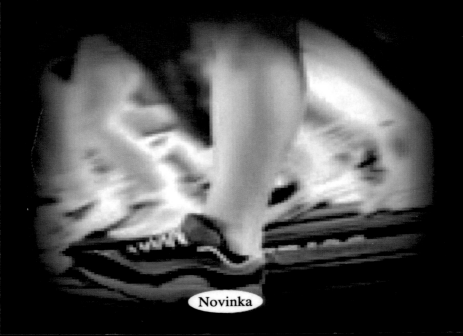

Novinka

GUIDE TO PHYSICAL FITNESS AND EXERCISE

GUIDE TO PHYSICAL FITNESS AND EXERCISE

PAMELA B. CARTER
EDITOR

Novinka Books
An imprint of Nova Science Publishers, Inc.
New York

For permission to use material from this book please contact us:
Telephone 631-231-7269; Fax 631-231-8175
Web Site: http://www.novapublishers.com

G-V481
.C34
2006
cop 1

NOTICE TO THE READER

The Publisher has taken reasonable care in the preparation of this book, but makes no expressed or implied warranty of any kind and assumes no responsibility for any errors or omissions. No liability is assumed for incidental or consequential damages in connection with or arising out of information contained in this book. The Publisher shall not be liable for any special, consequential, or exemplary damages resulting, in whole or in part, from the readers' use of, or reliance upon, this material.

Independent verification should be sought for any data, advice or recommendations contained in this book. In addition, no responsibility is assumed by the publisher for any injury and/or damage to persons or property arising from any methods, products, instructions, ideas or otherwise contained in this publication.

This publication is designed to provide accurate and authoritative information with regard to the subject matter covered herein. It is sold with the clear understanding that the Publisher is not engaged in rendering legal or any other professional services. If legal or any other expert assistance is required, the services of a competent person should be sought. FROM A DECLARATION OF PARTICIPANTS JOINTLY ADOPTED BY A COMMITTEE OF THE AMERICAN BAR ASSOCIATION AND A COMMITTEE OF PUBLISHERS.

Library of Congress Cataloging-in-Publication Data:
Available Upon Request

ISBN: 1-59454-737-8

LC Control Number

2007   272661

Published by Nova Science Publishers, Inc. ✦ *New York*

CONTENTS

PREFACE

Evidence is mounting each day that exercise is crucial not only for fitness but for overall health and even in battles against specific diseases such as Parkinson's, arthritis and heart disease. Exercise is basically free except for time and it is that which many people are determined not to part with. This book offers a guide to exercise and fitness originally published by the Presidents' Council on Fitness. Here it is excerpted, reorganized and indexed for access and combined with related relevant information.

In: Guide to Physical Fitness and Exercise   ISBN 1-59454-737-8
Editor: Pamela B. Carter, pp. 1-81   © 2006 Nova Science Publishers, Inc.

Chapter 1

A GUIDE TO EXERCISE[*]

National Institute on Aging

Dear Friends:

You are never too old to get in shape. I am often asked what I've done over the years to stay in shape. At different times, I have engaged in many different activities. When I was in school I played football and basketball. The Marine Corps provided its own unique brand of physical training or PT. While in the space program and for many years afterwards, I jogged to stay in shape. And my wife Annie and I have enjoyed hiking and skiing over the years. Most of all, I have always valued staying active in one way or another.

From my involvement with NASA, both in the Mercury program and with the Shuttle Mission STS-95, I have become keenly aware of the effect that weightlessness can have on the human body. Without the effect of gravity, astronauts' muscles and bones begin to deteriorate while they're in space. A number of other changes occur to the astronauts in orbit — from which they recover upon their return — that also happen as part of the natural aging process right here on Earth. For one, osteoporosis sets in. These same things can happen to us if we maintain a sedentary lifestyle. This is especially true as we get older.

The good news is that exercise is just a step away. I am pleased to recommend *Exercise: A Guide from the National Institute on Aging* as an excellent manual for anyone who wants to take those first steps toward an active lifestyle. The scientists and doctors at the National Institute on Aging

---

[*] Extracted from http://weboflife.nasa.gov/exerciseandaging/home.html

at the National Institutes of Health collaborated to produce this top-notch book. This guide contains valuable information about how exercise and proper nutrition are crucial for staying healthy as we age and provides useful tips on establishing and maintaining a regular exercise program.

In my case, I had to make accommodations to my advancing years by modifying my exercise regime. In the past, I was an ardent jogger, but as I got older my doctor said that the impact of running was putting too much stress on my knees and other joints. He suggested that I take up speed walking instead. Along with that, I do some weight lifting and stretching. So now I still get a great workout, but by doing exercise that is appropriate for my age and physical condition. This guide will help you do the same.

I hope you will read this book and follow its suggestions. We can all enjoy healthy and productive senior years by heeding these recommendations.

Senator John Glenn

INTRODUCTION

Welcome to one of the healthiest things you can do for yourself. Exercise! Regular exercise and physical activity are very important to the health and abilities of older people. In fact, studies suggest that *not* exercising is risky behavior. That is why we wrote this book. We are the National Institute on Aging, part of the National Institutes of Health, and our research is aimed at improving the health of older people.

For the most part, when older people lose their ability to do things on their own, it doesn't happen just because they have aged. More likely, it is because they have become inactive. Older inactive adults lose ground in four areas that are important for staying healthy and independent: endurance, strength, balance, and flexibility.

Fortunately, research suggests that you can maintain or at least partly restore these four areas through exercise — or through everyday physical activities (walking briskly or gardening, for example) that accomplish some of the same goals as exercise. What may seem like very small changes resulting from exercise and physical activity can have a big impact.

Getting Past the Barriers

You may be reluctant to start exercising, even though you've heard that it's one of the healthiest things you can do. You may be afraid that physical activity will harm you; or you might think you have to join a gym or buy expensive equipment in order to exercise. Or, you may feel embarrassed to exercise because you think it's for younger people or for people who look great in gym clothes. You may think exercise is only for people who are able to do things like jogging.

In fact, just about every older adult can safely do some form of physical activity at little or no cost. And you don't have to exercise in a public place or use expensive equipment, if you don't want to.

Even household chores can improve your health. The key is to increase your physical activity, by exercising and by using your own muscle power.

Who Can Exercise?

Studies show that, in the long term, older adults in all age groups hurt their health far more by not exercising than by exercising. As a rule, older people should stay as physically active as they can.

Section 2 of this book explains that there are certain situations in which you should check with your doctor before starting to exercise. You will also find out about a couple of conditions that prohibit exercise. More than likely, though, reading Section 2 will reassure you, but if you still have any doubts about exercise, talk to your doctor before you start.

About this Chapter

"The good news... is that people can benefit from even moderate levels of physical activity."
Surgeon General of the United States

The first three sections of this book explain what exercise and physical activity can do for you, how to exercise safely, and how to stay motivated to exercise. If you already know the material in Sections 1 and 2 — for example, if your doctor already has talked to you about the benefits of exercise and has advised you how to exercise safely — skip to the summary at the end of each section to make sure that you aren't missing any important information, then go to Section 3, which discusses motivation.

Fact: Together, lack of exercise and poor diet are the second-largest underlying cause of death in the United States. (Smoking is the #1 cause.)

Section 4 is a "how-to" section. It shows how to exercise to improve or maintain endurance, strength, balance, and flexibility. You certainly aren't restricted to these exercises. We show you these examples to help you get started.

Section 5 also is a "howto" section. It gives examples of ways you can check your progress. The last section is about nutrition. Each section summary lists important points to remember.

"I walk, garden, and do housework. Exercise keeps me limber. Most people don't think I'm my age."
Darrell Randall, 81, Washington, D.C.

At the end of the book, you will find resources to contact for more information about exercise and special programs for older exercisers. Some of the resources are for people with diseases or disabilities. You will also find charts to record your progress and a form you can fill out and send to us after you have been exercising for at least a month. We will send you a National Institute on Aging certificate that acknowledges your commitment to improving your health through exercise.

A Word about Words

Terms used to discuss exercise can be confusing. We want to explain a few key words used in this book.

- You probably have heard the term "aerobics" or "aerobic exercises." We call them "endurance exercises" or "endurance activities." These activities increase your heart rate and breathing for an extended period of time.
- The term "cardiovascular" refers to your heart and circulatory systems.
- The word "frailty" has more than one meaning. We use it here to mean the physical condition that results, in part, from severe muscle loss — the kind of muscle loss seen in people who have been inactive for

many years. Frail people have severe loss of strength and often cannot perform everyday tasks.

- We frequently use the word "independence"; in this book, it means older adults' ability to live and do things on their own. Being independent doesn't necessarily mean doing things alone; it means being able to do for yourself, in your everyday tasks and your leisure activities, to the greatest extent possible.

- Exercises that build muscle have a variety of names, including "strength-training," "resistance-training," "weight-training," or "weight-lifting." In this book, we call them "muscle-building" or "strength" exercises.

- What is considered a physical activity and what is considered an exercise? A physical activity is any voluntary body movement that burns calories. Exercise is physical activity that follows a planned format. It's done with repeated movements, with the goal of improving or keeping up one or more specific areas of physical fitness.

His Garden Grows

"My exercise focus is on gardening," Arthur Canfield, 83, of Fairfax, Virginia, told us. "I hate the thought of exercise for exercise's sake. I've never done that," he said.

Mr. Canfield grew up close to the soil. He remembers driving horses pulling hay, sometimes all day, and carrying water down to the garden on his uncle's farm. His wife grew up in a family that made its living in the wholesale florist trade, so she, too, understood gardens.

Mr. Canfield and his wife brought their lifelong affinity for gardening with them into their marriage. When they settled in Fairfax, near Mr. Canfield's job as an economist, the house they bought had about an acre of land, and they worked it — and worked it. "I didn't want to be deskbound when I became a bureaucrat. That's when I decided to become a serious gardener," he said.

Gardening, Mr. Canfield told us, gives you an opportunity to exercise every part of your body and get satisfaction out of it at the same time. He said that gardening does more than build muscle and endurance. "You have to keep your balance. You're reaching up to prune trees, bending over to check your tomato plants. The actual energy output at any given moment may not amount to much, but your whole system is participating the whole time," he said. It adds up.

Mr. Canfield lives on his own and drives himself wherever he needs to go. He works in his garden 3 or 4 hours every day.

"It's got to be fun," he said. "I like to work what I do into a rhythmic pattern. Splitting wood, chopping down trees — the rhythmic pattern of exercise is like music. You're absolutely a free spirit. You forget about it as you're doing it."

Mr. Canfield thinks that the idea of exercise sounds grim to most people — as though they have to do it, because there will be penalties if they don't.

"But raking leaves is not something you should dread; it's a joyous thing. In New England, it's as much of an event as sugaring-off the maples; it's the center of things for a while," he said.

He wants to give other older adults the following message about increasing their physical activity: "Once they start, they'll see that it builds on itself. It feels so good."

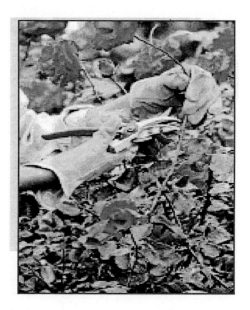

1. WHAT CAN EXERCISE DO FOR ME?

Most people know that exercise is good for them. Somehow, though, older adults have been left out of the picture — until recently. Today a new picture is emerging from research: Older people of different physical conditions have much to gain from exercise and from staying physically active. They also have much to lose if they become physically *in*active.

Exercise isn't just for older adults in the younger age range, who live independently and are able to go on brisk jogs, although this book is for them, too. Researchers have found that exercise and physical activity also can improve the health of people who are 90 or older, who are frail, or who have the diseases that seem to accompany aging. Staying physically active and exercising regularly can help prevent or delay some diseases and disabilities as people grow older. In some cases, it can improve health for older people who already have diseases and disabilities, if it's done on a long-term, regular basis.

What Kinds of Activities Improve Health and Ability?

Four types of exercises help older adults gain health benefits:

Endurance exercises increase your breathing and heart rate. They improve the health of your heart, lungs, and circulatory system. Having more endurance not only helps keep you healthier; it can also improve your stamina for the tasks you need to do to live and do things on your own — climbing stairs and grocery shopping, for example. Endurance exercises also may delay or prevent many diseases associated with aging, such as diabetes, colon cancer, heart disease, stroke, and others, and reduce overall death and hospitalization rates.

Strength exercises build your muscles, but they do more than just make you stronger. They give you more strength to do things on your own. Even very small increases in muscle can make a big difference in ability, especially for frail people.

Fact: More than two-thirds of older adults don't engage in regular physical activity.

Strength exercises also increase your metabolism, helping to keep your weight and blood sugar in check. That's important because obesity and diabetes are major health problems for older adults. Studies suggest that strength exercises also may help prevent osteoporosis.

Balance exercises help prevent a common problem in older adults: falls. Falling is a major cause of broken hips and other injuries that often lead to disability and loss of independence. Some balance exercises build up your leg muscles; others require you to do simple activities like briefly standing on one leg.

Flexibility exercises help keep your body limber by stretching your muscles and the tissues that hold your body's structures in place. Physical therapists and other health professionals recommend certain stretching exercises to help patients recover from injuries and to prevent injuries from happening in the first place. Flexibility also may play a part in preventing falls.

Which Ones Should I Do, and How Much Should I Do?

Some types of exercise improve just one area of health or ability. More often, though, an exercise has many different benefits.

In other words, exercise as much as you can. It's best to increase both the types and amounts of exercises and physical activities you do. Gradually build up to include: endurance, strength, balance, and flexibility exercises. (We show you how in Section 4.)

Now that you have read about all the benefits of exercise, we hope you are enthusiastic about getting started. However, it's important to start at a level you can manage and work your way up gradually.

For one thing, if you do too much too quickly, you can damage your muscles and tissues, and that can keep you on the sidelines. For another, your enthusiasm needs to last a lifetime. The benefits of exercise and physical activity come from making them a permanent habit. Start with one or two types of exercises that you can manage and that you really can fit into your schedule, then add more as you adjust to ensure that you will stick with it.

"Exercise is like a savings account. The more you put in, the more you're going to get out of it."
Ron Ekovich, 61, Leesville, South Carolina

How much you exercise depends on you and on your unique situation. For some, muscle-building exercise might mean pushing more than a hundred pounds of weight at the local gym to keep your legs in shape for hiking or jogging. For others, it might mean lifting 1-pound weights to strengthen your arm muscles enough to use a washcloth. That might mean the dignity that comes from being able to wash yourself, instead of having someone else do it for you. The goal is to improve from wherever you are right now.

Some people are reluctant to start exercising because they are afraid it will be too strenuous. Researchers have found that you don't have to do strenuous exercises to gain health benefits; moderate exercises are effective, too. (You will read more about the difference between vigorous and moderate exercises later in this book.)

Fact: Many people 90 and older who have become physically frail from inactivity can more than double their strength through simple exercises in a fairly short time. For some, that can mean the difference between getting up from a chair by themselves or depending on someone to help them. In one study, some people 80 and older progressed from using walkers to using canes after doing simple muscle-building exercises for just 10 weeks.

How Much Physical Activity is Enough?

Everyday physical activities can accomplish some of the same goals as exercise. But just how much should you do to get health benefits?

We can't always give you answers, yet, but we can give examples of what researchers have found out. For instance, bus and taxi drivers, who are physically *in*active, have a higher rate of heart disease than men in other occupations. And studies show that people who remain physically active have a lower death rate than people who don't.

In another study, researchers measured muscle strength in 75-year-olds who regularly did tasks like housework and gardening and in 75-year-olds who were inactive. Five years later they found that the active people kept more of their strength than did the inactive people.

While we can't yet tell you exactly how much everyday physical activity you should get to gain specific health benefits, the message of these studies is clear: Whatever your age, stay physically active!

In Section 4, we give you specific types and amounts of exercises to do. They can help you not only maintain your current levels of strength and fitness, but also help you build them up. Our examples also might encourage you to exercise muscles and joints that you have stopped using or that you use less often without even realizing it.

Section 1 Summary

Research suggests that growing older does not mean you have to lose your strength and ability to do everyday tasks and the things you enjoy doing. But an inactive lifestyle does mean that you probably will lose some of your strength and ability, and that you will be at higher risk for diseases and disabilities. Fortunately, even many frail people can improve their health and independence by increasing their physical activity.

Challenging exercises and physical activities done regularly can help many older adults improve their health, even when done at a moderate level. They may prevent or delay a variety of diseases and disabilities associated with aging.

Four types of exercises are important:

(1) Endurance activities increase heart rate and breathing for extended periods of time. They improve the health of the heart, lungs, and circulatory system, and help prevent or delay some diseases.
(2) Strength exercises make older adults strong enough to do the things they need to do and the things they like to do.
(3) Balance exercises help prevent falls, a major cause of disability in older adults.
(4) Stretching helps keep the body limber and flexible.

Every Crisis is an Opportunity

Dr. Andrew Puckett is a busy man with an impressive list of titles after his name. The 60-year-old associate dean for medical education at Duke University, in Durham, North Carolina, has a Ph.D. in adult education and a minor in clinical psychology, and he has been a counselor for years. He also has Parkinson's disease, a chronic condition that causes muscles to tremble and become rigid. He was diagnosed with it a few years ago.

Has his chronic condition slowed down his activities? It doesn't appear that way. In addition to his regular activities, 2 years ago, Dr. Puckett volunteered to take part in a study of how stretching exercises affect people with Parkinson's disease. He enjoyed the feeling of stretching so much that he kept doing the exercises after the 10-week study ended, and now does them at least 3 days a week for 40 minutes at a time.

It's not yet clear whether or not stretching exercises have an effect on Parkinson's disease specifically, but it's very clear to Dr. Puckett that they have helped him feel better overall.

"I literally feel so much better from doing the exercises," he told us. "I'm more flexible than I've been in 20 years. Stretching has given me so much ease of movement. It's a fluid feeling," he said. In addition, Dr. Puckett finds that stretching exercises give him a sense of well-being. He likens it to the "runner's high" that some joggers experience.

Dr. Puckett noted another positive aspect of his stretching exercises: the feeling that he is nurturing himself. He described it as a secure feeling; a feeling that he is doing something good for himself.

Another motivator for keeping up with his stretching exercises is "the fear of being stiff and rigid; bent over. I want to keep that from happening," he told us.

Besides working at the university, Dr. Puckett splits his own firewood, plays tennis, gardens, mows his lawn with a push mower, and walks a mile or more at least 3 days a week.

"But people shouldn't feel that physical activity has to be some super-human or highly disciplined effort," he said. "I don't want them to be scared off from the idea of exercising. I think once they experience how much better they feel, they'll want to keep on doing it. It has so many built-in benefits."

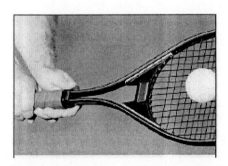

2. IS IT SAFE FOR ME TO EXERCISE?

"Too old" and "too frail" are not, in and of themselves, reasons to prohibit physical activity. In fact, there aren't very many health reasons to keep older adults from becoming more active.

Most older people think they need their doctor's approval to start exercising. That's a good idea for some people. Your doctor can talk to you not only about whether it's all right for you to exercise but also about what can be gained from exercise.

Chronic Diseases: Not Necessarily a Barrier

Chronic diseases can't be cured, but usually they can be controlled with medications and other treatments throughout a person's life. They are common among older adults, and include diabetes, cardiovascular disease (such as high blood pressure), and arthritis, among many others.

Traditionally, exercise has been discouraged in people with certain chronic conditions. But researchers have found that exercise can actually improve some chronic conditions in most older people, *as long as it's done when the condition is under control.*

Congestive heart failure (CHF) is an example of a serious chronic condition common in older adults. In people with CHF, the heart can't empty its load of blood with each beat, resulting in a backup of fluid throughout the body, including the lungs. Disturbances in heart rhythm also are common in CHF. Older adults are hospitalized more often for this disease than for any other.

No one is sure why, but muscles tend to waste away badly in people with CHF, leaving them weak, sometimes to the point that they can't perform everyday tasks. No medicine has a direct muscle-strengthening effect in people with CHF, but muscle-building exercises (lifting weights, for example) can help them improve muscle strength.

Having a chronic disease like CHF probably doesn't mean you can't exercise. But it does mean that keeping in touch with your doctor is important if you do exercise. For example, some studies suggest that endurance exercises, like brisk walking, may improve how well the heart and lungs work in people with CHF, *but only in people who are in a stable phase of the disease.* People with CHF, like those with most chronic diseases, have periods when their disease gets better, then worse, then better again, off and on. The same endurance exercises that might help people in a stable phase of CHF could be very harmful to people who are in an unstable phase; that is, when they have fluid in their lungs or an irregular heart rhythm.

If you have a chronic condition, you need to know how you can tell whether your disease is stable; that is, when exercise would be OK for you and when it wouldn't.

Chances are good that, if you have a chronic disease, you see a doctor regularly

> "At our age, you have to exercise. I just feel that exercise enhances our state of living. You can walk, for example. You don't have to be out there competing with everybody."
> Jeanette Chamberlain, 73, Silver Spring, Maryland

(if you don't, you should, for many reasons). Talk with your doctor about symptoms that mean trouble — a flare-up, or what doctors call an acute phase or exacerbation of your disease. If you have CHF, you know by now that the acute phase of this disease should be taken very, very seriously. You should *not* exercise when warning symptoms of the acute phase of CHF, or any other chronic disease, appear. It could be dangerous.

But you and your doctor also should discuss how you feel when you are free of those symptoms — in other words, stable; under control. This is the time to exercise.

Diabetes is another chronic condition common among older people. Too much sugar in the blood is a hallmark of diabetes. It can cause damage throughout the body. Exercise can help your body "use up" some of the damaging sugar.

The most common form of diabetes is linked to physical *in*activity. In other words, you are less likely to get it in the first place, if you stay physically active.

> "I feel my day isn't complete without some physical activity. I know I do miss it on the days that I don't do it."
> Harriet Erickson, 72, Durham, North Carolina

If you do have diabetes and it has caused changes in your body — cardiovascular disease, eye disease, or changes in your nervous system, for example — check with your doctor to find out what exercises will help you and whether you should avoid certain activities. If you take insulin or a pill that helps lower your blood sugar, your doctor might need to adjust your dose so that your blood sugar doesn't get too low.

Your doctor might find that you don't have to modify your exercises at all, if you are in the earlier stages of diabetes or if your condition is stable.

If you are a man over 40 or a woman over 50, check with your doctor first if you plan to start doing *vigorous*, as opposed to moderate, physical activities. Vigorous activity could be a problem for people who have "hidden" heart disease — that is, people who have heart disease but don't know it because they don't have any symptoms.

How can you tell if the activity you plan to do is vigorous? There are a couple of ways. If the activity makes you breathe hard and sweat hard (if you tend to sweat, that is), you can consider it vigorous. Charts in Section 4 explain more about how to tell if your exercise is moderate or vigorous.

Fact: The Surgeon General has issued a report warning people — including older adults — that physical *in*activity is a major risk to their health.

If you have had a heart attack recently, your doctor or cardiac rehabilitation therapist should have given you specific exercises to do. Research has shown that exercises done as part of a cardiac rehabilitation program can improve fitness and even reduce your risk of dying. If you didn't get instructions, call your doctor to discuss exercise before you begin increasing your physical activity.

For some conditions, vigorous exercise is dangerous and should not be done, even in the absence of symptoms. Be sure to check with your physician before beginning any kind of exercise program if you have:

- abdominal aortic aneurysm, a weakness in the wall of the heart's major outgoing artery (unless it has been surgically repaired or is so small that your doctor tells you that you can exercise vigorously)
- critical aortic stenosis, a narrowing of one of the valves of the heart.

Most older adults, regardless of age or condition, will do just fine in increasing their physical activity. You might want to show your doctor this book, to open the door to discussions about exercise.

Section 2 Summary

Contrary to traditional thinking, regular exercise helps, not hurts, most older adults. Older people become sick or disabled more often from **not** exercising than from exercising. Those who have chronic diseases, or risk factors for them, may actually improve with regular exercise, but should check with their doctor before increasing their physical activity.

There are few reasons to keep older adults from increasing their physical activity, and "too old" and "too frail" aren't among them.

If you plan to work your way up to a vigorous level, check with your doctor first if you are a man over 40 or a woman over 50. Also check with your doctor first if you have any of the conditions listed under "Checkpoints."

Your doctor or cardiac rehabilitation specialist can give you guidelines for physical activity if you have had a heart attack recently. Controlled exercise usually is an important part of long-term heart-attack recovery.

People with conditions called "abdominal aortic aneurysm" or "critical aortic stenosis" should not exercise unless their physicians tell them they can.

Almost all older adults, regardless of age or condition, can safely improve their health and independence through exercise and physical activity.

Checkpoints

You have already read about precautions you should take if you have a chronic condition. Other circumstances require caution, too. You shouldn't exercise until checking with a doctor if you have:

- chest pain
- irregular, rapid, or fluttery heart beat
- severe shortness of breath
- significant, ongoing weight loss that hasn't been diagnosed
- infections, such as pneumonia, accompanied by fever
- fever, which can cause dehydration and a rapid heart beat
- acute deep-vein thrombosis (blood clot)
- a hernia that is causing symptoms
- foot or ankle sores that won't heal
- joint swelling
- persistent pain or a problem walking after you have fallen
- certain eye conditions, such as bleeding in the retina or detached retina. Before you exercise after a cataract or lens implant, or after laser treatment or other eye surgery, check with your physician.

Building Strength, Inner and Outer

At the age of 70, Harriet Erickson, of Durham, North Carolina, tended her husband through the terminal illness that took his life. The loss of her husband hurt her deeply. "It was a horrible time for me. I wasn't in very good shape, physically or emotionally," she told us.

Soon after, Ms. Erickson volunteered to take part in a study of exercise for older adults. Participants did endurance and flexibility exercises. Erickson liked how the exercises made her feel and kept doing them at home after the study ended.

She has this to say about exercise: "It's made my life a lot better. I was slumped over. Now, I stand up straight, and I can look the world right in the eye. I don't intend to stop. I know what a difference it has made for me."

Researchers have shown that exercise can help relieve anxiety and stress, and can improve mood. They just aren't able to tell you that in quite the same way Ms. Erickson can.

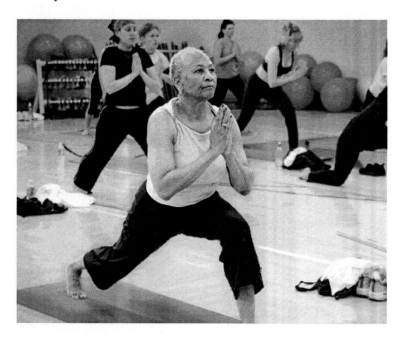

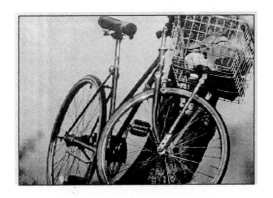

3. HOW TO KEEP GOING

"Definitely NOT!" That's what 75-year-old Emma King told us when we asked her if she ever intended to stop exercising. Ms. King lives in Durham, North Carolina, and has taken long walks at least 4 or 5 days a week, for years. Recently, she took part in a study of exercise for older adults and added stretching to her weekly routine. "I can really tell the difference if I miss 2 or 3 days. I don't know what it would be like not to exercise," she said.

For many older adults, motivation to keep exercising and doing physical activities isn't a problem. They say that regular physical activity makes them feel so much better that it would be hard to stop.

Others say that, while physical activity makes them feel better, a little extra motivation helps them get going. For example, Georgia Burnette, 68, of Amherst, New York, told us that she used to put on headphones and listen to recorded books borrowed from the library to make her 40-minute walks more interesting. Now, she mall-walks for an hour, 5 days a week, with a friend. Having that companionship is a good motivator, says Ms. Burnette.

We have included this section on motivation because physical activity needs to be a regular, permanent habit to produce benefits like those listed in Section 1. So does staying motivated!

Recording your scores and watching them improve can be an excellent motivator to exercise, and we have included charts at the end of this booklet so you can do that. But don't get discouraged if you see that your scores have improved by only a few seconds or just one or two lifts of a weight. In terms of real-life benefits, those slight improvements are multiplied many times over as you include them in your everyday activities. You incorporate that extra little bit of endurance and strength into everything you do, and it adds up to a lot.

But no matter how enthusiastic you are about exercise, there may be times when you need extra motivation. It's common for beginning exercisers, especially those who are frail, to make fast progress at first. You might get discouraged when the improvements you were making taper off at times.

Sticking with it: What Works

According to the U.S. Surgeon General's report, you are more likely to keep doing physical activities if you:

- think that, overall, you will benefit from them
- include activities you enjoy
- feel you can do the activities correctly and safely
- have regular access to the activities
- can fit the activities into your daily schedule
- feel that the activities don't impose financial or social costs you aren't willing to take on
- have few negative consequences from doing your activities (such as injury, lost time, or negative peer pressure)

In other words, set yourself up to succeed right from the start. Choose realistic goals, learn to do the exercises correctly and safely, and chart your progress to see your improvement.

These leveling-off periods are normal. Often, they mean that it's time to gradually make your activities more challenging. If you have any doubts about whether you are doing the right things to progress, check the guidelines listed under each type of exercise in Section 4, or check with your doctor or a qualified fitness professional (see page 23).

When you need extra motivation, try the following:

- Ask someone to be your exercise buddy. Many older adults agree that having someone to exercise with helps keep them going.
- Follow Georgia Burnette's advice: Listen to recorded books or music while you do endurance activities.
- Set a goal, and decide on a reward you will get when you reach it.

- Give yourself physical activity homework assignments for the next day or the next week.
- Think of your exercise sessions as appointments, and mark them on your calendar.
- Keep a record of what you do and of your progress. Understand that there will be times that you don't show rapid progress and that you are still benefiting from your activities during those times.
- Plan ahead for travel, bad weather, and house guests. For example, an exercise video can help you exercise indoors when the weather is bad.

"Everybody has to find their own way to exercise. They have to embrace it and make it work for them."

Georgia Burnette, 68, Amherst, New York

Let us Acknowledge Your Efforts

When it comes to motivation, the first month is crucial. If you can increase your physical activity for a month and keep going after that, you will have passed a critical landmark. It's a good sign that you are on your way to making exercise and physical activity regular, life-long habits.

We want to give you credit for that. If you increase your physical activity for more than a month, send us the form at the end of this book. We will send you a National Institute on Aging certificate acknowledging your commitment.

Section 3 Summary

Starting with one or two types of exercises or physical activities and a schedule that you really can manage, then adding more as you adjust, is one way of ensuring that you will keep exercising. You are also more likely to keep exercising if you feel you can do your exercises correctly and safely, feel that they fit into your schedule, and don't feel that they result in negative experiences, such as financial burdens or lost time.

Just knowing that physical activity can improve your health and abilities can be enough to keep you exercising, but you might need extra motivation sometimes. For those times, try exercising with a friend, listening to music, charting your progress, marking your calendar for exercise sessions, giving yourself exercise "assignments" ahead of time, and rewarding yourself when you achieve your goals.

Overall, your fitness should improve. If it doesn't, review the instructions on how to progress in Section 4.

If you stick with your exercises for more than a month, it's a good sign that you are on your way to making it a permanent habit. If you would like acknowledgment of your efforts, fill out the form at the end of this book, and we will send you a National Institute on Aging certificate.

Finding a Qualified Fitness Professional

Most older people can exercise just fine on their own, without advice from a fitness instructor. Some have special needs and may want to consult a professional. If you decide to seek advice, how can you tell whom to trust? Anyone can call himself or herself a fitness professional, and many people do — but that doesn't always mean they have the training to help older people exercise safely and effectively.

Instructors who aren't trained to work with older adults, specifically, might not be aware of their needs. For example, they might not know that certain conditions or medications can change older people's heart rates or that people with osteoporosis risk spine fractures if they do some types of forward-bending exercises incorrectly.

A number of professionals are familiar with the special physical needs of older people. Doctors who specialize in sports medicine are highly qualified to help you exercise the right way. So are professionals who have a college degree in exercise physiology. They can help you start an exercise program tailored to your needs, build it up to your best possible level, then show you how to continue safely on your own.

Physical therapists also are qualified to design exercise plans for older people, especially those who have conditions affecting their muscles and skeletal systems, or nervous-system conditions that affect their muscles. Some physical therapists take special training for a certification in geriatrics.

The American College of Sports Medicine (ACSM) also trains and certifies people to work with older adults. The ACSM is made up of health professionals and scientists with an interest in fitness. ACSM-certified fitness instructors work in a variety of settings; for example, you might find them leading hospital-based exercise programs for older adults, working with older people in exercise studies, or working as personal trainers.

Cardiologists can advise you on how to improve your cardiovascular system through endurance exercise. Orthopedic doctors can help you understand how to prevent injuries to your muscles, bones, and other structures.

Many hospitals and health plans now have wellness centers that offer exercise programs. Some colleges and universities hold special exercise classes for older adults or conduct studies on exercise for older people. It's likely that the fitness instructors hired by these organizations are carefully screened and are qualified to teach you how to exercise correctly. Try calling them to find a fitness professional in your area.

If you do consult a fitness instructor, ask for his or her credentials. Any instructor who is qualified to work with older people is likely to be proud of his or her credentials and will be happy to share them with you. Also ask about expense. Costs vary, and insurance plans differ as to what kinds of services they will cover.

Making it Work

There are lots of ways to increase your physical activity. Exercising at home is just one of them, and we feature it here because it's within the reach of most older people. Or, you might decide to follow Phyllis Wendahl's example, instead, and do something different.

Ms. Wendahl is 85 years old and lives in the small town of Bothell, Washington. On the phone, she sounds much younger. She is a widow and lives on her Social Security income, and, like many older adults, she won't let her kids spoil her as much as they would like to. She would rather do things on her own.

That's why, when she was scouting around for a fitness club where she could use strength-building equipment, she bargained the owner down to a monthly fee that she felt she could afford — $25 a month for unlimited use.

"Look, I know that not everybody is as bold as I am about that kind of thing," Ms. Wendahl told us. Nonetheless, she has some advice for older adults who are thinking about going to a fitness center: "They don't need to feel self-conscious about going to the club. The owner of my club holds me up as an example now."

Ms. Wendahl said that she has always been active, but never as much as she is now. She began doing aerobic exercises in her 70s, moved on to water aerobics, and most recently to strength-building and stretching 3 times a week. She lives on he own and drives herself wherever she needs to go.

After 6 months of endurance and strength exercises, measurements showed that Ms. Wendahl was able to perform household tasks — carrying groceries, making her bed, and transferring laundry — more quickly. She could also carry more weight.

"It has just done me a world of good," she said of her physically active lifestyle. "My family is so thrilled and proud of me," she added.

She wants older adults who read this book to know that, when it comes to exercise and physical activity, "there's always something within someone's capabilities. There's no reason older people need to be sitting in a rocking chair."

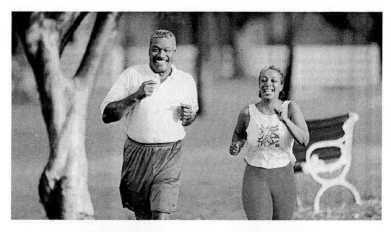

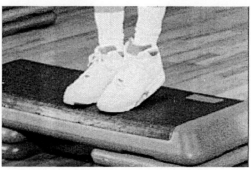

4. SAMPLE EXERCISES

Many different physical activities can improve your health and independence. Whether you choose to do the exercises shown in this section or other activities that accomplish the same goals, gradually work your way up to include endurance, strength, balance, and stretching exercises.

Here are some points to keep in mind as you begin increasing your activity:

- If you stop exercising for several weeks and then return, start out at about half the effort you were putting into it when you stopped, then gradually build back up. Some of the effects of endurance and muscle-building exercises deteriorate within 2 weeks if these activities are cut back substantially, and benefits may disappear altogether if they aren't done for 2 to 8 months.
- When an exercise calls for you to bend forward, bend from the hips, not the waist. If you keep your entire back and shoulders straight as you bend forward, that will help ensure that you are bending the right way, from the hips. If you find your back or shoulders humping in any spot as you bend forward, that's a sign that you are bending incorrectly, from the waist. Bending from the waist may cause spine fractures in some people with osteoporosis.
- It's possible to combine exercises. For example, regular stair-climbing sessions improve endurance and strengthen leg muscles at the same time.

How Hard Should I Exercise?

We can't tell you exactly how many pounds to lift or how steep a hill you should climb to reach a moderate or vigorous level of exercise, because what is easy for one person might be strenuous for another. It's different for different people.

We can, however, provide some advice based on scientific research: Listen to your body. The level of effort you feel you are putting into an activity is likely to agree with actual physical measurements. In other words, if your body tells you that the exercise you are doing is moderate, measurements of how hard your heart is working would probably show that it really is working at a moderate level. During moderate activity, for instance, you can sense that you are challenging yourself but that you aren't near your limit.

One way you can estimate how hard to work is by using the Borg Category Rating Scale, shown on the next page. It was named after Gunnar Borg, the scientist who developed it. The numbers on the left of the scale don't indicate how many times or how many minutes you should do an activity; they help you describe how hard you feel you are working.

For **endurance activities**, you should **gradually** work your way up to **level 13** — the feeling that you are working at a somewhat hard level. Some people might feel that way when they are walking on flat ground; others might feel that way when they are jogging up a hill. Both are right. Only *you* know how hard your exercise feels to you.

Strength exercises are higher on the Borg scale. **Gradually** work your way up to **level 15 to 17** — hard to very hard — to build muscle effectively. You can tell how hard an effort you are making by comparing it to your maximum effort. How hard does your current effort feel compared to when you are lifting the heaviest weight you can lift? Once you start exerting more than a moderate amount of effort in your muscle-building exercises, your strength is likely to increase quickly.

As your body adapts and you become more fit, you can gradually keep making your activities more challenging. You might find, for example, that walking on a flat surface used to feel like you were working at level 13 on the Borg scale, but now you have to walk up a mild hill to feel like you are working at level 13. Later, you might find that you need to walk up an even steeper slope to feel that you are working at level 13.

The Borg scale is simple to use. But if your level of effort doesn't match the numbers you see on the Borg scale — for example, if you think you are doing the exercises correctly, but you aren't progressing or you are exhausted by your effort — check with a fitness professional (see page 23). These experts are likely to understand the science that went into developing the Borg scale, and they can teach you how to match your level of effort with the right number on the scale.

The Borg Category Rating Scale		
Least effort		
6		
7	very, very light	
8		
9	very light	
10		
11	fairly light	ENDURANCE TRAINING
12		
13	somewhat hard	
14		
15	hard	STRENGTH TRAINING
16		
17	very hard	
18		
19	very, very hard	
20		
Maximum effort		

How to Improve Your Endurance

Endurance exercises are any activity — walking, jogging, swimming, raking — that increases your heart rate and breathing for an extended period of time.

How Much, How Often

- **Build up your endurance gradually,** starting out with as little as 5 minutes of endurance activities at a time, if you need to.
- Starting out at a lower level of effort and working your way up gradually is especially important if you have been inactive for a long time. **It may take months to go from a very long-standing sedentary lifestyle to doing some of the activities suggested in this section.**
- Your goal is to work your way up, eventually, to a moderate-to-vigorous level that increases your breathing and heart rate. **It should feel somewhat hard** to you (level 13 on the Borg scale).
- Once you reach your goal, you can divide your exercise into sessions of **no less than 10 minutes at a time,** if you want to, as

long as they add up to a total of a minimum of 30 minutes at the end of the day. Doing less than 10 minutes at a time won't give you the desired cardiovascular and respiratory system benefits. (The exception to this guideline is when you are just beginning to do endurance activities.)

- Your goal is to build up to **a minimum of 30 minutes of endurance exercise on most or all days of the week.** More often is better, and every day is best.

Safety

- Endurance activities should not make you breathe so hard that you can't talk. They should not cause dizziness or chest pain.
- Do a little light activity before and after your endurance exercise session, to warm up and cool down (example: easy walking).
- Stretch *after* your endurance activities, when your muscles are warm.
- As you get older, your body may become less likely to trigger the urge to drink when you need water. In other words, you may need water, but you won't feel thirsty.
- Be sure to drink liquids when you are doing any activity that makes you lose fluid through sweat. The rule of thumb is that, by the time you notice you are thirsty, you are already somewhat dehydrated (low on fluid). This guideline is important year-round, but is especially important in hot weather, when dehydration is more likely. If your doctor has asked you to limit your fluids, be sure to check with him or her before increasing the amount of fluid you drink while exercising. Congestive heart failure and kidney disease are examples of chronic diseases that often require fluid restriction.
- Older adults can be affected by heat and cold more than other adults. In extreme cases, exposure to too much heat can cause heat stroke, and exposure to very cold temperatures can lead to hypothermia (a dangerous drop in body temperature). If you are exercising outdoors, dress in layers so you can add or remove clothes as needed.
- Use safety equipment to prevent injuries. For example, wear a helmet for bicycling, and wear protective equipment for activities like skiing and skating. If you walk or jog, wear stable shoes made for that purpose.

Tips on How to Gauge Your Effort

Here are some informal guidelines you can use to estimate how much effort you are putting into your endurance activities.

- Talking doesn't take much effort during moderate activity. During vigorous activity, talking is difficult.
- If you tend to perspire, you probably won't sweat during light activity (except on hot days). You will sweat during vigorous or sustained moderate activity.
- Your muscles may get a rubbery feeling after vigorous activity, but not after moderate activity.
- One doctor who specializes in exercise for older adults tells her patients this about how hard they should work during endurance activities: "If you can't talk while you're exercising, it's too difficult. If you can sing a song from an opera, it's too easy!"

Progressing

When you are ready to progress, build up the amount of time you spend doing endurance activities first; then build up the difficulty of your activities later. Example: First, gradually increase your time to 30 minutes over several days to weeks (or even months, depending on your condition) by walking longer distances, then start walking up steeper hills or walking more briskly.

Examples of Endurance Activities

Examples of activities that are moderate for the average older adult are listed below.

Moderate
- Swimming
- Bicycling
- Cycling on a stationary bicycle
- Gardening (mowing, raking)
- Walking briskly on a level surface
- Mopping or scrubbing floor
- Golf, without a cart
- Tennis (doubles)
- Volleyball
- Rowing

- Dancing

The following are examples of vigorous activities.

Vigorous
- Climbing stairs or hills
- Shoveling snow
- Brisk bicycling up hills
- Tennis (singles)
- Swimming laps
- Cross-country skiing
- Downhill skiing
- Hiking
- Jogging

How to Improve Your Strength

Even very small changes in muscle size can make a big difference in strength, especially in people who already have lost a lot of muscle. An increase in muscle that's not even visible to the eye can be all it takes to improve your ability to do things like get up from a chair or climb stairs.

Your muscles are active even when you are sleeping. Their cells are still doing the routine activities they need to do to stay alive. This work is called metabolism, and it uses up calories. That can help keep your weight in check, even when you are asleep!

About Strength Exercises

To do most of the following strength exercises, you need to lift or push weights, and gradually you need to increase the amount of weight you use. You can use the hand and ankle weights sold in sporting-goods stores, or you can use things like emptied milk jugs filled with sand or water, or socks filled with beans and tied shut at the ends.

There are many alternatives to the exercises shown here. For example, you can buy a resistance band (it looks like a giant rubber band, and stretching it helps build muscle) at a sporting-goods store to do other types of strength exercises. Or you can use the special strength-training equipment at a fitness center.

How Muscles Work

What makes your muscles look bigger when you flex them — when you "make a muscle" with your biceps, for example?

Muscle cells contain long strands of protein lying next to each other. When you want your muscles to move, your brain signals your nerves to stimulate them. A chemical reaction in your muscles follows, causing the long strands of protein to slide toward and over each other, shortening the length of your muscle cells. When you "make a muscle" and you see your muscle bunch up and bulge, you are actually watching it shorten as the protein strands slide over each other.

When you do challenging muscle-building exercises on a regular basis, the bundles of protein strands inside your muscle cells grow bigger.

How Much, How Often

- Do strength exercises for all of your major muscle groups **at least twice a week.** Don't do strength exercises of the same muscle group on any 2 days in a row.
- Depending on your condition, you might need to start out using as little as 1 or 2 pounds of weight, or no weight at all. The tissues that bind the structures of your body together need to adapt to strength exercises.
- **Use a minimum of weight the first week,** then gradually add weight. Starting out with weights that are too heavy can cause injuries.
- Gradually add a challenging amount of weight in order to benefit from strength exercises. If you don't challenge your muscles, you won't benefit from strength exercises. (The "Progressing" section on page 34 will tell you how.)
- When doing a strength exercise, do **8 to 15 repetitions in a row.** Wait a minute, then do another set of 8 to 15 repetitions in a row of the same exercise. (Tip: While you are waiting, you might want to stretch the muscle you just worked or do a different strength exercise that uses a different set of muscles).
- Take **3 seconds to lift or push a weight** into place; **hold the position for 1 second,** and take **another 3 seconds to lower the weight.** Don't let the weight drop; lowering it slowly is very important.

- It should feel somewhere between hard and very hard (15 to 17 on the Borg scale) for you to lift or push the weight. It should not feel very, very hard. If you can't lift or push a weight 8 times in a row, it's too heavy for you. Reduce the amount of weight. If you can lift a weight more than 15 times in a row, it's too light for you. Increase the amount of weight.
- Stretch after strength exercises, when your muscles are warmed up. If you stretch before strength exercises, be sure to warm up your muscles first (through light walking and arm pumping, for example).

> ## Practice Sitting Straight
>
> Sit or stand with your shoulders back, but not pinched, and hold this position while you take slow, deep breaths. You can do this anytime.

Safety

- **Don't hold your breath during strength exercises.** Breathe normally. Holding your breath while straining can cause changes in blood pressure. This is especially true for people with cardiovascular disease.
- If you have had a hip repair or replacement, check with your surgeon before doing lower-body exercises.
- If you have had a hip replacement, don't cross your legs, and don't bend your hips farther than a 90-degree angle.
- Avoid jerking or thrusting weights into position. That can cause injuries. Use smooth, steady movements.
- Avoid "locking" the joints in your arms and legs in a tightly straightened position. (A tip on how to straighten your knees:
- Tighten your thigh muscles. This will lift your kneecaps and protect them.)
- Breathe out as you lift or push, and breathe in as you relax. For example, if you are doing leg lifts, breathe out as you lift your leg, and breathe in as you lower it. This may not feel natural at first, and you probably will have to think about it as you are doing it for awhile.

- Muscle soreness lasting up to a few days and slight fatigue are normal after muscle-building exercises, but exhaustion, sore joints, and unpleasant muscle pulling aren't. The latter symptoms mean you are overdoing it.
- None of the exercises you do should cause pain. The range within which you move your arms and legs should never hurt.

Progressing

- Gradually increasing the amount of weight you use is crucial for building strength.
- When you are able to lift a weight between 8 to 15 times, you can increase the amount of weight you use at your next session.
- Here is an example of how to progress gradually: Start out with a weight that you can lift only 8 times. Keep using that weight until you become strong enough to lift it 12 to 15 times. Add more weight so that, again, you can lift it only 8 times. Use this weight until you can lift it 12 to 15 times, then add more weight. Keep repeating.

Fact: Although they might not notice it as it happens, most people lose 20 to 40 percent of their muscle tissue as they get older. Strength exercise can at least partly restore muscle and strength.

Sarcopenia: A Word You are Likely to Hear More About

We know that muscle-building exercises can improve strength in most older adults, but many questions remain about muscle loss and aging. Researchers want to know, for example, if factors other than a sedentary lifestyle contribute to muscle loss. Does age itself cause changes in the muscles of older people? Is muscle loss related to changes in hormones or nutrition? The answers to these questions may lead to ways of helping us keep our strength as we age.

In this book, we use the word "frailty" to describe the loss of muscle and strength often seen in older people, because it's a word that most people are familiar with. However, a better word to use is "sarcopenia" (pronounced sar - ko - PEEN - ya). It means not only the loss of muscle and strength but also the decreased quality of muscle tissue often seen in older adults. You are likely to hear more about sarcopenia in the future since it's a very active area of research.

Examples of Strength Exercises

Arm Raise
Strengthens shoulder muscles.

1.   Sit in armless chair with your back supported by back of chair.
2.   Keep feet flat on floor even with your shoulders.
3.   Hold hand weights straight down at your sides, with palms facing inward.
4.   Raise both arms to side, shoulder height.
5.   Hold the position for 1 second.
6.   Slowly lower arms to sides. Pause.
7.   Repeat 8 to 15 times.
8.   Rest; then do another set of 8 to 15 repetitions.

Chair Stand
Strengthens muscles in abdomen and thighs. Your goal is to do this exercise without using your hands as you become stronger.

1.   Place pillows on the back of chair.
2.   Sit toward front of chair, knees bent, feet flat on floor.
3.   Lean back on pillows in half-reclining position. Keep your back and shoulders straight throughout exercise.
4.   Raise upper body forward until sitting upright, using hands as little as possible (or not at all, if you can). Your back should no longer lean against pillows.
5.   Slowly stand up, using hands as little as possible.
6.   Slowly sit back down. Pause.
7.   Repeat 8 to 15 times.
8.   Rest; then do another set of 8 to 15 repetitions.

Biceps Curl
Strengthens upper-arm muscles.

1.   Sit in armless chair with your back supported by back of chair.
2.   Keep feet flat on floor even with your shoulders.
3.   Hold hand weights straight down at your sides, with palms facing inward.
4.   Slowly bend one elbow, lifting weight toward chest. (Rotate palm to face shoulder while lifting weight.)

5. Hold position for 1 second.
6. Slowly lower arm to starting position. Pause.
7. Repeat with other arm.
8. Alternate arms until you have done 8 to 15 repetitions with each arm.
9. Rest; then do another set of 8 to 15 alternating repetitions.

Plantar Flexion
Strengthens ankle and calf muscles. Use ankle weights, if you are ready.

1. Stand straight, feet flat on floor, holding onto a table or chair for balance.
2. Slowly stand on tiptoe, as high as possible.
3. Hold position for 1 second.
4. Slowly lower heels all the way back down. Pause.
5. Do the exercise 8 to 15 times.
6. Rest; then do another set of 8 to 15 repetitions.

Variation: As you become stronger, do the exercise standing on one leg only, alternating legs for a total of 8 to 15 times on each leg. Rest; then do another set of 8 to 15 alternating repetitions.

Triceps Extension
(If your shoulders aren't flexible enough to do this exercise, see alternative "Dip" exercise.)
Strengthens muscles in back of upper arm. Keep supporting your arm with your hand throughout the exercise.

1. Sit in chair with your back supported by back of chair.
2. Keep feet flat on floor even with shoulders.
3. Hold a weight in one hand. Raise that arm straight toward ceiling, palm facing in.
4. Support this arm, below elbow, with other hand.
5. Slowly bend raised arm at elbow, bringing hand weight toward same shoulder.
6. Slowly straighten arm toward ceiling.
7. Hold position for 1 second.
8. Slowly bend arm toward shoulder again. Pause.
9. Repeat the bending and straightening until you have done the exercise 8 to 15 times.

10. Repeat 8 to 15 times with your other arm.
11. Rest; then do another set of 8 to 15 alternating repetitions.

Alternative "Dip" Exercise for Back of Upper Arm

This pushing motion will strengthen your arm muscles even if you aren't yet able to lift yourself up off of the chair. Don't use your legs or feet for assistance, or use them as little as possible.

1. Sit in chair with armrests.
2. Lean slightly forward, keep your back and shoulders straight.
3. Grasp arms of chair. Your hands should be level with trunk of body or slightly farther forward.
4. Tuck feet slightly under chair, heels off the ground, weight on toes and balls of feet.
5. Slowly push body off of chair using arms, not legs.
6. Slowly lower back down to starting position. Pause.
7. Repeat 8 to 15 times.
8. Rest; then do another set of 8 to 15 repetitions.

Knee Flexion

Strengthens muscles in back of thigh. Use ankle weights, if you are ready.

1. Stand straight holding onto a table or chair for balance.
2. Slowly bend knee as far as possible. Don't move your upper leg at all; bend your knee only.
3. Hold position for 1 second.
4. Slowly lower foot all the way back down. Pause.
5. Repeat with other leg.
6. Alternate legs until you have done 8 to 15 repetitions with each leg.
7. Rest; then do another set of 8 to 15 alternating repetitions.

Hip Flexion

Strengthens thigh and hip muscles. Use ankle weights, if you are ready.

1. Stand straight to the side or behind a chair or table, holding on for balance.
2. Slowly bend one knee toward chest, without bending waist or hips.
3. Hold position for 1 second.
4. Slowly lower leg all the way down. Pause.

5. Repeat with other leg.
6. Alternate legs until you have done 8 to 15 repetitions with each leg.
7. Rest; then do another set of 8 to 15 alternating repetitions.

Shoulder Flexion
Strengthens shoulder muscles.

1. Sit in armless chair with your back supported by back of chair.
2. Keep feet flat on floor even with your shoulders.
3. Hold hand weights straight down at your sides, with palms facing inward.
4. Raise both arms in front of you (keep them straight and rotate so palms face upward) to shoulder height.
5. Hold position for 1 second.
6. Slowly lower arms to sides. Pause.
7. Repeat 8 to 15 times.
8. Rest; then do another set of 8 to 15 repetitions.

Knee Extension
Strengthens muscles in front of thigh and shin. Use ankle weights, if you are ready.

1. Sit in chair. Only the balls of your feet and your toes should rest on the floor. Put rolled towel under knees, if needed, to lift your feet. Rest your hands on your thighs or on the sides of the chair.
2. Slowly extend one leg in front of you as straight as possible.
3. Flex foot to point toes toward head.
4. Hold position for 1 to 2 seconds.
5. Slowly lower leg back down. Pause.
6. Repeat with other leg.
7. Alternate legs until you have done 8 to 15 repetitions with each leg.
8. Rest; then do another set of 8 to 15 alternating repetitions.

Hip Extension
Strengthens buttock and lower-back muscles. Use ankle weights, if you are ready.

1. Stand 12 to 18 inches from a table or chair, feet slightly apart.
2. Bend forward at hips at about 45-degree angle; hold onto a table or chair for balance.

3. Slowly lift one leg straight backwards without bending your knee, pointing your toes, or bending your upper body any farther forward.
4. Hold position for 1 second.
5. Slowly lower leg. Pause.
6. Repeat with other leg.
7. Alternate legs until you have done 8 to 15 repetitions with each leg.
8. Rest; then do another set of 8 to 15 alternating repetitions.

Side Leg Raise
Strengthens muscles at sides of hips and thighs. Use ankle weights, if you are ready.

1. Stand straight, directly behind table or chair, feet slightly apart.
2. Hold onto a table or chair for balance.
3. Slowly lift one leg 6-12 inches out to side. Keep your back and both legs straight. Don't point your toes outward; keep them facing forward.
4. Hold position for 1 second.
5. Slowly lower leg. Pause.
6. Repeat with other leg.
7. Alternate legs until you have done 8 to 15 repetitions with each leg.
8. Rest; then do another set of 8 to 15 alternating repetitions.

How to Improve Your Balance

Each year, U.S. hospitals have 300,000 admissions for broken hips, and falling is often the cause of those fractures. Balance exercises can help you stay independent by helping you avoid the disability — often permanent — that may result from falling.

As you will see, there is a lot of overlap between strength and balance exercises; very often, one exercise serves both purposes.

About Strength/Balance Exercises
Any of the lower-body exercises for strength shown in the previous strength section also are balance exercises. They include plantar flexion, hip flexion, hip extension, knee flexion, and side leg raise. Just do your regularly scheduled strength exercises, and they will improve your balance at the same time. Also do the knee-extension exercise, which helps you keep your balance by increasing muscle strength in your upper thighs.

Safety

- Don't do more than your regularly scheduled strength-exercise sessions to incorporate these balance modifications.
- Remember that doing strength exercises too often can do more harm than good.
- Simply do your strength exercises, and incorporate these balance techniques as you progress.

Progressing

These exercises can improve your balance even more if you add the following modifications: Note that these exercises instruct you to hold onto a table or chair for balance. Hold onto the table with only one hand. As you progress, try holding on with only one fingertip. Next, try these exercises without holding on at all. If you are very steady on your feet, move on to doing the exercises using no hands, with your eyes closed. Have someone stand close by if you are unsteady.

Examples of Strength/Balance Exercises

Plantar Flexion

Plantar flexion is already included in your strength exercises. When doing your strength exercises, add these modifications to plantar flexion as you progress: Hold table with one hand, then one fingertip, then no hands; then do exercise with eyes closed, if steady.

1. Stand straight; hold onto a table or chair for balance.
2. Slowly stand on tip toe, as high as possible.
3. Hold position for 1 second.
4. Slowly lower heels all the way back down. Pause.
5. Repeat 8 to 15 times.
6. Rest; then do another set of 8 to 15 repetitions.
7. Add modifications as you progress.

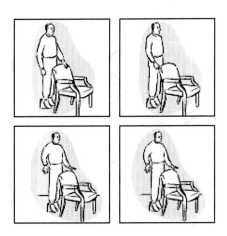

Knee Flexion

Do knee flexion as part of your regularly scheduled strength exercises, and add these modifications as you progress: Hold table with one hand, then one fingertip, then no hands; then do exercise with eyes closed, if steady.

1.   Stand straight; hold onto a table or chair for balance.
2.   Slowly bend knee as far as possible, so foot lifts up behind you.
3.   Hold position for 1 second.
4.   Slowly lower foot all the way back down. Pause.
5.   Repeat with other leg.
6.   Alternate legs until you have done 8 to 15 repetitions with each leg.
7.   Rest; then do another set of 8 to 15 alternating repetitions.
8.   Add modifications as you progress.

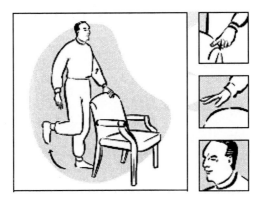

Hip Flexion

Do hip flexion as part of your regularly scheduled strength exercises, and add these modifications as you progress: Hold table with one hand, then one fingertip, then no hands; then do exercise with eyes closed, if steady.

1. Stand straight; hold onto a table or chair for balance.
2. Slowly bend one knee toward chest, without bending waist or hips.
3. Hold position for 1 second.
4. Slowly lower leg all the way down. Pause.
5. Repeat with other leg.
6. Alternate legs until you have done 8 to 15 repetitions with each leg.
7. Rest; then do another set of 8 to 15 alternating repetitions.
8. Add modifications as you progress.

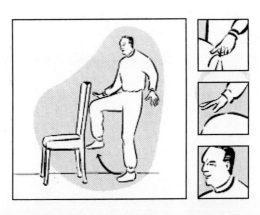

Hip Extension

Do hip extension as part of your regularly scheduled strength exercises, and add these modifications as you progress: Hold table with one hand, then one fingertip, then no hands; then do exercise with eyes closed, if steady.

1. Stand 12 to 18 inches from a table or chair, feet slightly apart.
2. Bend forward at hips at about 45-degree angle; hold onto a table or chair for balance.
3. Slowly lift one leg straight backwards without bending your knee, pointing your toes, or bending your upper body any farther forward.
4. Hold position for 1 second.
5. Slowly lower leg. Pause.
6. Repeat with other leg.
7. Alternate legs until you have done 8 to 15 repetitions with each leg.
8. Rest; then do another set of 8 to 15 alternating repetitions.
9. Add modifications as you progress.

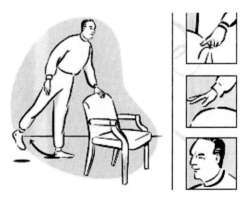

Side Leg Raise

Do leg raise as part of your regularly scheduled strength exercises, and add these modifications as you progress: Hold table with one hand, then one fingertip, then no hands; then do exercise with eyes closed, if steady.

1. Stand straight, directly behind table or chair, feet slightly apart.
2. Hold onto table or chair for balance.

3. Slowly lift one leg to side 6-12 inches out to side. Keep your back and both legs straight. Don't point your toes outward; keep them facing forward.
4. Hold position for 1 second.
5. Slowly lower leg all the way down. Pause.
6. Repeat with other leg.
7. Alternate legs until you have done 8 to 15 repetitions with each leg.
8. Rest; then do another set of 8 to 15 alternating repetitions.
9. Add modifications as you progress.

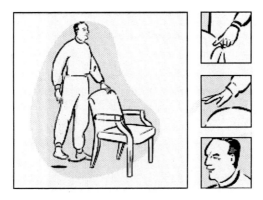

"Anytime, Anywhere" Balance Exercises

These types of exercises also improve your balance. You can do them almost anytime, anywhere, and as often as you like, as long as you have something sturdy nearby to hold onto if you become unsteady.

Examples:

*   Walk heel-to-toe. Position your heel just in front of the toes of the opposite foot each time you take a step. Your heel and toes should touch or almost touch. (See illustration.)
*   Stand on one foot (for example, while waiting in line at the grocery store or at the bus stop). Alternate feet.
*   Stand up and sit down without using your hands.

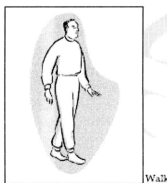

Walk heel-to-toe.

How to Improve Your Flexibility

Stretching exercises give you more freedom of movement to do the things you need to do and the things you like to do. Stretching exercises alone can improve your flexibility, but they will not improve your endurance or strength.

How Much, How Often

- Stretch after you do your regularly scheduled strength and endurance exercises.
- If you can't do endurance or strength exercises for some reason, and stretching exercises are the only kind you are able to do, do them at least 3 times a week, for at least 20 minutes each session.
- Do each stretching exercise 3 to 5 times at each session.
- Slowly stretch into the desired position, as far as possible without pain, and hold the stretch for 10 to 30 seconds. Relax, then repeat, trying to stretch farther.

Safety

- If you have had a hip replacement, check with your surgeon before doing lower body exercises.
- If you have had a hip replacement, don't cross your legs or bend your hips past a 90-degree angle.

- Always warm up before stretching exercises (do them after endurance or strength exercises, for example; or, if you are doing only stretching exercises on a particular day, do a little bit of easy walking and arm-pumping first). Stretching your muscles before they are warmed up may result in injury.
- Stretching should never cause pain, especially joint pain. If it does, you are stretching too far and you need to reduce the stretch so that it doesn't hurt.
- Mild discomfort or a mild pulling sensation is normal.
- Never "bounce" into a stretch; make slow, steady movements instead. Jerking into position can cause muscles to tighten, possibly resulting in injury.
- Avoid "locking" your joints into place when you straighten them during stretches. Your arms and legs should be straight when you stretch them, but don't lock them in a tightly straight position. You should always have a very small amount of bending in your joints while stretching.

Progressing

You can progress in your stretching exercises; the way to know how to limit yourself is that stretching should never hurt. It may feel slightly uncomfortable, but not painful. Push yourself to stretch farther, but not so far that it hurts.

Examples of Stretching Exercises

Hamstrings

Stretches muscles in the back of the thigh.

1. Sit sideways on bench or other hard surface (such as two chairs placed side by side).
2. Keep one leg stretched out on bench, straight, toes pointing up.
3. Keep other leg off of bench, with foot flat on floor.
4. Straighten back.
5. If you feel a stretch at this point, hold the position for 10 to 30 seconds.
6. If you don't feel a stretch, lean forward from hips (not waist) until you feel stretching in leg on bench, keeping back and shoulders

straight. Omit this step if you have had a hip replacement, unless surgeon/therapist approves.

7. Hold position for 10 to 30 seconds.
8. Repeat with other leg.
9. Repeat 3 to 5 times on each side.

Alternative Hamstrings Stretch

Stretches muscles in the back of the thigh.

1. Stand behind chair, holding the back of it with both hands.
2. Bend forward from the hips (not waist), keeping back and shoulders straight at all times.
3. When upper body is parallel to floor, hold position for 10 to 30 seconds. You should feel a stretch in the backs of your thighs.
4. Repeat 3 to 5 times.

Calves

Stretches lower leg muscles in two ways: with knee straight and knee bent.

1. Stand with hands against wall, arms outstretched and elbows straight.
2. Keeping your left knee slightly bent, toes of right foot slightly turned inward, step back 1-2 feet with right leg, heel, and foot flat on floor. You should feel a stretch in your calf muscle, but you shouldn't feel uncomfortable. If you don't feel a stretch, move your foot farther back until you do.
3. Hold position for 10 to 30 seconds.
4. Bend knee of right leg, keep heel and foot flat on floor.
5. Hold position for another 10 to 30 seconds.
6. Repeat with left leg.
7. Repeat 3 to 5 times for each leg.

Ankles

Stretches front ankle muscles.

1. Remove your shoes. Sit toward the front edge of a chair and lean back, using pillows to support your back.
2. Stretch legs out in front of you.

3. With your heels still on the floor, bend ankles to point feet toward you.
4. Bend ankles to point feet away from you.
5. If you don't feel the stretch, repeat with your feet slightly off the floor.
6. Hold the position for 1 second.
7. Repeat 3 to 5 times.

Triceps Stretch
Stretches muscles in back of upper arm.

1. Hold one end of a towel in right hand.
2. Raise and bend right arm to drape towel down back. Keep your right arm in this position, and continue holding onto the towel.
3. Reach behind your lower back and grasp bottom end of towel with left hand.
4. Climb left hand progressively higher up towel, which also pulls your right arm down. Continue until your hands touch, or as close to that as you can comfortably go.
5. Reverse positions.
6. Repeat each position 3 to 5 times.

Wrist Stretch
Stretches wrist muscles.

1. Place hands together, in praying position.
2. Slowly raise elbows so arms are parallel to floor, keeping hands flat against each other.
3. Hold position for 10 to 30 seconds.
4. Repeat 3 to 5 times.

About Floor Exercises

Most of the remaining exercises are done on the floor and stretch some very important muscle groups. If you are afraid to lie on the floor to exercise because you think you won't be able to get back up, consider using the buddy system to do these. Find a buddy who will be able to help you.

Knowing the right way to get into a lying position on the floor and to get back up also may be helpful. If you have had a hip replacement, check with your surgeon before using the following method. If you have osteoporosis, check with your doctor first.

To Get into a Lying Position
- Stand next to a very sturdy chair that won't tip over (put chair against wall for support if you need to).
- Put your hands on the seat of the chair.
- Lower yourself down on one knee.
- Bring the other knee down.
- Put your left hand on the floor and lean on it as you bring your left hip to the floor.
- Your weight is now on your left hip.
- Straighten your legs out.
- Lie on your left side.
- Roll onto your back.
- Note: You don't have to use your left side. You can use your right side, if you prefer.

To Get Up from a Lying Position
- Roll onto your left side.
- Use your right hand, placed on the floor at about the level of your ribs, to push your shoulders off the floor.
- Your weight is on your left hip.
- Roll forward, onto your knees, leaning on your hands for support.
- Lean your hands on the seat of the chair you used to lie down.
- Lift one of your knees so that one leg is bent, foot flat on the floor.
- Leaning your hands on the seat of the chair for support, rise from this position.
- Note: You don't have to use your left side; you can reverse positions, if you prefer.

Quadriceps
Stretches muscles in front of thighs.

1. Lie on side on the floor. Your hips should be lined up so that one is directly above the other one.
2. Rest head on pillow or hand.
3. Bend knee that is on top.

4. Reach back and grab heel of that leg. If you can't reach your heel with your hand, loop a belt over your foot and hold belt ends.
5. Gently pull that leg until front of thigh stretches.
6. Hold position for 10 to 30 seconds.
7. Reverse position and repeat.
8. Repeat 3 to 5 times on each side. If the back of your thigh cramps during this exercise, stretch your leg and try again, more slowly.

Double Hip Rotation

Stretches outer muscles of hips and thighs. Don't do this exercise if you have had a hip replacement, unless your surgeon approves.

1. Lie on floor on your back, knees bent and feet flat on the floor.
2. Keep shoulders on floor at all times.
3. Keeping knees bent and together, gently lower legs to one side as far as possible without forcing them.
4. Hold position for 10 to 30 seconds.
5. Return legs to upright position.
6. Repeat toward other side.
7. Repeat 3 to 5 times on each side.

Single Hip Rotation

Stretches muscles of pelvis and inner thigh. Don't do this exercise if you have had a hip replacement, unless your surgeon approves.

1. Lie on your back on floor, knees bent and feet flat on the floor.
2. Keep shoulders on floor throughout exercise.
3. Lower one knee slowly to side, keeping the other leg and your pelvis in place.
4. Hold position for 10 to 30 seconds.
5. Bring knee back up slowly.
6. Repeat with other knee.
7. Repeat 3 to 5 times on each side.

Shoulder Rotation

Stretches shoulder muscles.

1. Lie flat on floor, pillow under head, legs straight. If your back bothers you, place a rolled towel under your knees.

2. Stretch arms straight out to side. Your shoulders and upper arms will remain flat on the floor throughout this exercise.
3. Bend elbows so that your hands are pointing toward the ceiling. Let your arms slowly roll backwards from the elbow. Stop when you feel a stretch or slight discomfort, and stop immediately if you feel a pinching sensation or a sharp pain.
4. Hold position for 10 to 30 seconds.
5. Slowly raise your arms, still bent at the elbow, to point toward the ceiling again. Then let your arms slowly roll forward, remaining bent at the elbow, to point toward your hips. Stop when you feel a stretch or slight discomfort.
6. Hold position for 10 to 30 seconds.
7. Alternate pointing above head, then toward ceiling, then toward hips. Begin and end with pointing-above-head position.
8. Repeat 3 to 5 times.

Neck Rotation

Stretches neck muscles.

1. Lie on the floor with a phone book or other thick book under your head.
2. Slowly turn head from side to side, holding position each time for 10 to 30 seconds on each side. Your head should not be tipped forward or backward, but should be in a comfortable position. You can keep your knees bent to keep your back comfortable during this exercise.
3. Repeat 3 to 5 times.

Section 4 Summary

- Build up to all exercises and activities gradually, especially if you have been inactive for a long time.
- Once you have built up to a regular schedule, include endurance, strength, balance, and stretching exercises.
- If you have to stop exercising for more than a few weeks, start at half the effort when you resume, then build back up to where you were.
- When bending forward, always keep back and shoulders straight to ensure that you are bending from the hips, not the waist.

- If you have had a hip replacement, check with your surgeon before doing lower body exercises.

Endurance

- To build stamina, you can do specific exercises, like walking or jogging, or any activity that raises your heart rate and breathing for extended periods of time.
- Do at least 30 minutes of endurance activities on most or all days of the week.
- If you prefer, divide your 30 minutes into shorter sessions of no less than 10 minutes each.
- The more vigorous the exercise, the greater the benefits.
- Warm up and cool down with a light activity, such as easy walking.
- Activities shouldn't make you breathe so hard you can't talk. They shouldn't cause dizziness or chest pain.
- When you are ready to progress, first increase the amount of time, then the difficulty, of your activity.
- Stretch after endurance exercises.

Strength

- Do strength exercises for all your major muscle groups at least twice a week, but not for the same muscle group on any 2 days in a row.
- Gradually increasing the amount of weight you use is the most important part of strength exercise.
- Start with a low amount of weight (or no weight) and increase it gradually.
- When you are ready to progress, first increase the number of times you do the exercise, then increase the weight at a later session.
- Do an exercise 8 to 15 times; rest a minute and repeat it 8 to 15 more times.
- Take 3 seconds to lift and 3 seconds to lower weights. Never jerk weights into position.
- If you can't lift a weight more than 8 times, it's too heavy; if you can lift it more than 15 times, it's too light.
- Don't hold your breath while straining.
- These exercises may make you sore at first, but they should never cause pain.
- Stretch after strength exercises.

Balance

- Add the following modifications to your regularly scheduled lower-body strength exercises: As you progress, hold onto the table or chair with one hand, then one finger, then no hands. If you are steady on your feet, progress to no hands and eyes closed. Ask someone to watch you the first few times, in case you lose your balance.
- Don't do extra strength exercises to add these balance modifications. Simply add the modifications to your regularly scheduled strength exercises.
- Another way to improve your balance is through "anytime, anywhere" balance exercises. One example: Balance on one foot, then the other, while waiting for the bus. Do as often as desired.

Stretching

- Stretching exercises may help keep you limber.
- Stretching exercises alone will not improve endurance or strength.
- Do stretching exercises after endurance and strength exercises, when your muscles are warm.
- If stretching exercises are the only kind of exercise you are able to do, do them at least 3 times a week, up to every day. Always warm up your muscles first.
- Do each exercise 3 to 5 times at each session.
- Hold the stretched position for 10 to 30 seconds.
- Total session should last 15 to 30 minutes.
- Move slowly into position; never jerk into position.
- Stretching may cause mild discomfort, but should not cause pain.

Enjoying Retirement

Until he was 48 years old, Ron Ekovich, of Leesville, South Carolina, smoked a pack of cigarettes every day. Looking to the future made him decide to quit.

"I figured I had to make some changes in my life if I was going to enjoy my retirement," he told us.

Needless to say, Mr. Ekovich, who is now 61 years old, no longer smokes. He works out with strength-building equipment 3 days a week, and he carries his own bag of clubs on the 3 days a week that he plays golf.

And he stretches. "If I had to choose the most important thing you can do as you get older, it would be stretching. It helps keep you selfsufficient," he said. Mr. Ekovich was only halfjoking when he gave an example: When his back itches, he said, he's able to just reach back and scratch it. This example might seem funny... unless you aren't able to scratch your own back.

"The more physical activity you get the better you feel. The achievement makes you feel great emotionally, and it makes you feel good physically," he said.

Mr. Ekovich also cites a person's outlook as an important component of physical activity and exercise. "The only thing that limits people's ability to achieve their goals is themselves," he said. He recently finished shoveling about 10 tons of earth — that's 20,000 pounds — to make a new garden for his wife.

5. How Am I Doing?

There are ways to tell when it's time to move ahead in your activities, and we have mentioned some of them in the preceding section. For example, when you can lift a weight more than 15 times, you know it's time to add more weight in your strength exercises. And when endurance activities no longer feel somewhat hard to you, it's time to exercise a little longer, then to add a little more difficulty, like walking up steeper hills.

As you progress, you can do some simple tests, shown in this section, that will tell you just how far you have come. These tests also can help you assess how fit you are before you start exercising. After that, try them again every month. Record your scores each time, so you can see your improvement the next time you test yourself.

You might be interested in doing these tests for a couple of reasons. For one, most people make rapid progress soon after they start exercising, and you might find the improvement you see in your scores after just a month encouraging.

For another, these tests are a good way of letting you know if you really are progressing. Although it's normal for your improvement to slow down at times, your test scores should get better overall (unless you have reached your goal and are maintaining your current level).

If you are not in condition to do these tests right now, keep working on your current exercises and activities until you are. Whether you are testing or actually exercising, your pace should never make you feel dizzy, lightheaded, or nauseated, and you shouldn't feel pain. If you have a chronic medical condition, or are at risk of developing one, follow the guidelines in Section 2 before testing yourself.

❶ Endurance

See how far you can walk in exactly 6 minutes. Write down how far you walked (in feet, blocks, laps, miles, number of times you walked up and down a long hallway, or whatever is convenient for you). Do this test every month. As your endurance improves, you should find that you can walk farther in 6 minutes.

❷ Lower-Body Power

Time yourself as you walk up a flight of stairs (at least 10 steps) as fast as you safely can. Record your score. Repeat the test, using the same stairs, one month later. It should take you less time.

❸ Strength

Each time you do your strength exercises, use the chart in the back of this book to record how much weight you lift and how many times you lift that weight. Another chart shows how much more weight you can lift, and how many more times you can lift it, compared to the month before.

❹ Balance

Time yourself as you stand on one foot, without support, for as long as possible (stand near something sturdy to hold onto, in case you lose your balance). Record your score. Repeat the test while standing on the other foot. Test yourself again in one month. The amount of time you can stand on one foot should increase.

Fact: When astronauts come back to earth after extended space missions, they sometimes can't walk or perform other physical activities very well, at first. Because the weightlessness of space makes it possible for astronauts to push and pull objects without effort, their muscles become weak. Back on earth, the same principle applies to the muscles of sedentary older adults: If you don't use them, you lose them. The good news is that, at any age, almost any older adult —or astronaut — can improve strength through exercise.

Section 5 Summary

This section describes simple tests to see how you are progressing. They measure endurance, lower-body power, strength, and balance. Do the tests before you begin increasing your physical activity, to establish a baseline measurement. Repeat the tests each month. If you test yourself more often, you are not likely to see improvement, and that may discourage you. On the other hand, watching your scores improve every month can be very encouraging.

Be sure to use the safety guidelines listed for the exercises shown in Sections 2 and 4 when you do these tests.

You might not be able to complete the tests shown in this section, at first. That means you aren't ready yet. Try again after a month of exercises and physical activities.

More than One Way

"I want to walk young — I think exercise does that for you. You feel better. You feel younger." That's what Cecile Cress, 83, of Pueblo, Colorado, told us.

Ms. Cress used to ride her bicycle everywhere, up and down the hilly roads of her town, to get where she needed to go. She recently retired from her job as a librarian.

Ms. Cress stopped riding her bike when she found that it was hard for her to get started going up steep hills after traffic had stopped for red lights, making it unsafe for her.

"The thing I thought was so great about bike riding is that, going up a hill, you just feel like your heart is really pushing your blood through those veins and arteries," she said.

She didn't have to give up that feeling entirely when she stopped riding her bike. At least 3 days a week, Ms. Cress does exercises, including endurance and stretching, with the help of two videos for older adults. She began doing that years ago, during the winter, when it was too icy to ride her bike.

To make up for the activity she would miss when she stopped bike riding, Ms. Cress began going to a rehabilitation center to use strength-building equipment to improve her muscles and balance. She could have gone to a fitness club instead of a rehabilitation center, but there wasn't one that suited her needs in her area. With a little creative thinking, she and her daughter came up with the idea of asking if she could use the weight room at a local rehab center, instead. "I knew I had to do something when I stopped riding my bike," she said.

There are seniors' aerobics groups in Ms. Cress' area, but their hours don't fit into her schedule. "I know seniors who are doing it, though, and they look great," she said.

She has a secret she would like to share with other older adults who would like to stay in shape: Don't stop buying new clothes. Ms. Cress said that occasionally buying something new is one of the things that keeps her inspired to stay fit. "It's important to have more pride in your appearance as you get older. It's good to keep your weight down," she said.

"I never have to diet," she added. "I watch what I eat, but I don't diet."

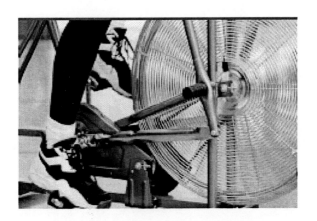

6. WHAT SHOULD I EAT?

Your body needs fuel for exercises and physical activities, and that fuel comes from food. Eating the right nutrients from a balanced diet helps build muscle and energy. But just what does "balanced diet" mean? What should you eat, and exactly how much of it should you eat?

The diagram shown on this page is the U.S. Department of Agriculture (USDA) food pyramid. If you use it as a guideline, you will be following a balanced diet. It tells you how many servings of each kind of food you should eat each day. We have also included a chart that shows you what, exactly, counts as one serving of each kind of food.

If you use the food pyramid as a guideline, you may also be helping to prevent or delay some of the diseases associated with growing older. For example, by cutting down on fats, you will be reducing your risk of getting cardiovascular diseases like high blood pressure. By increasing the amount of fruits and vegetables you eat, you will be lowering your risk of getting some types of cancer.

Looking at the guidelines, you will see that the biggest part of the calories you take in each day should come from grains, and the Some older adults are on restricted diets because of certain health conditions. Kidney disease is just one example of a condition that often requires restrictions of certain foods or fluids. If your doctor or nutritionist has asked you to follow a special diet, please follow his or her advice. smallest amount should come from fats, oils, and sweets. The guidelines put heavy emphasis on vegetables and fruits, and less on meat and dairy products.

Some older adults are on restricted diets because of certain health conditions. Kidney disease is just one example of a condition that often requires restrictions of certain foods or fluids. If your doctor or nutritionist has asked you to follow a special diet, please follow his or her advice.

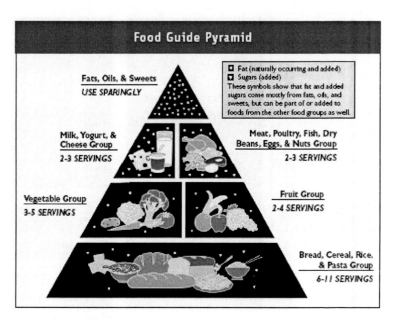

What is "A Serving"?

Grains
1 slice of bread
1/2 cup of cooked rice or pasta
1/2 cup of cooked cereal
1 ounce of ready-to-eat cereal

Fruits
1 piece of fruit
1 melon wedge
3/4 cup fruit juice
1/2 cup canned fruit
1/4 cup dried fruit

Vegetables
1/2 cup of chopped raw or cooked vegetables
1 cup of leafy raw vegetables

Milk, Yogurt, and Cheese
1 cup of milk or yogurt
1-1/2 to 2 ounces of cheese
Example: a 1-inch cube of hard cheese weighs about 1/2 ounce
Note: Buy low-fat or skim dairy products to avoid harmful fats.
Note: Some people have trouble digesting lactose, the sugar in milk products. If you have this problem, try eating yogurt with active cultures, low-fat cheese, or lactose-reduced milk. Pills and drops that help digest lactose also are available.

Meat, Poultry, Fish, Dry Beans, Eggs, and Nuts
1/2 cup of cooked beans, 1 egg, or 2 tablespoons of peanut butter make up 1/3 of a serving of this food group.

2-1/2 to 3 ounces of cooked lean meat, poultry, or fish make up one serving of this food group.

Examples: a slice of cooked, lean meat or poultry that is about 1/4- inch thick and measures 3 inches by 4 inches weighs about 2 ounces; a cooked, lean hamburger patty that weighs 3 ounces is about 3 inches across and 1/2- inch thick — about the size of a large mayonnaise jar lid.
Note: Before cooking, a patty this size weighs about 4 ounces.
Note: Half of a skinless, cooked chicken breast weighs about 3 ounces.
Note: Egg whites are a good source of protein, but egg yolks are high in fat and cholesterol. Consider discarding the yolk.
Note: Nuts are a good source of protein, but are high in fat.

Fats, Oils, and Sweets
The less fats, oils, and sweets you eat the better.

It's Really Not Hard to Eat a Balanced Diet

Do you look at the USDA food guidelines and think, "How in the world will I be able to follow them? I'd have a hard time just eating the 6 to 11 servings of grain I'm supposed to eat daily!" Take a look at the sample menu below, and you might change your mind. This menu provides the minimum amount recommended for each of the food groups. You might find that you are already eating a balanced diet and that you even have room to add more grains or fruits and vegetables.

Breakfast:
Western-style omelet (use egg whites or egg replacers and low-fat cheese)
Oven-baked hash-brown potatoes
Whole-grain toast and jelly
Small glass of fruit juice

Lunch:
Broiled salmon patty on a toasted whole-grain bun
Spinach
Rice
Fruit salad with low-fat or nonfat yogurt dressing

Dinner:
Pasta with tomato-andonion sauce, topped with low-fat parmesan cheese (lean meatballs optional)
Garlic bread
Salad with low-fat or nonfat dressing
Low-fat ice cream or frozen yogurt

The Big Picture

Often, people decide to exercise and eat a balanced diet because they want to control their weight. For many people, these healthy habits do result in weight loss…but that's only part of the big picture. Exercise and a healthy diet can help make you healthier. But they are just one part of becoming physically fit. Think about other lifestyle changes you can make, too. For example, smoking contributes to a variety of serious diseases and can keep you from exercising. So does excessive alcohol. Together, habits like exercise, a balanced diet, and giving up smoking will help you achieve what we wish for you: the best of health.

Section 6 Summary

A balanced diet is important for everyone, including older exercisers. To find out what "balanced diet" means, see the U.S. Department of Agriculture food-pyramid guidelines shown in this section. The guidelines say that the largest part of your calorie intake should be from grain-based foods; the next largest from vegetables and fruits; then fish, poultry, meats, and dairy products. The less fats, oils, and sweets you eat the better.

The best way to get the nutrients you need is through a healthy diet, not through expensive supplements that you might not need. Whole foods provide many nutrients we know about, and probably contain others that haven't been discovered. You might read or hear many convincing, scientific-sounding claims about nutritional supplements, such as megadoses of vitamins and minerals, but not all of them are based on fact. Some supplements may be helpful in certain situations, but others may cause harmful side effects. Before taking supplements of any kind, check with your doctor.

If your doctor or nutritionist has asked you to eat or avoid certain foods or fluids because of a medical condition, please follow his or her advice.

Supplements: Costly and Not Necessarily Helpful

Supplements are helpful for some older adults who can't eat all the nutrients they need — nutrients like vitamins and minerals. Recently, however, some new kinds of supplements have been appearing in stores even though they haven't been shown to improve health and their safety remains unproven.

A balanced diet is the best way for most older exercisers to get the nutrients they need. But some people in the marketing industry are doing a good job of convincing older people that they need expensive nutritional supplements, some of which haven't been shown to be helpful or safe and some of which most older people may not even need. Some of these claims give older adults the impression that certain supplements can restore youthful energy and strength.

For example, one persuasive clerk at a popular health-food store recently told an older shopper interested in exercise that she should buy certain supplements that cost about $70 a month to increase her energy and her ability to build muscles. The supplements included a protein powder and a vitamin-mineral pill containing the same ingredients as generic-brand vitamins, available at a fraction of the cost at drug stores, and some other substances not proven to build muscles or energy in older people.

This 75-year-old shopper had eaten an excellent diet based on the USDA food pyramid for years, and really didn't need these supplements.

No one likes to spend money needlessly, but for older adults on a limited income — Social Security, for example — unnecessary expenditures can deprive them of things they really do need (the money to buy whole foods rich in nutrients, for example). What's more, too much protein puts extra demands on the kidneys and can lower calcium levels. Although protein, vitamin, and mineral supplements are helpful to older people who truly need them, excessive doses can have harmful side effects.

A clerk at another health-food store told the same shopper that, if she planned to start exercising, she should buy a powder made of protein, vitamins, and minerals that cost $19 for a 10-serving bottle. Taken once a day, that comes out to about $60 a month. One of the reasons she needed this supplement, the clerk told her, was that it contained the mineral potassium, and "older people require more of that."

Taken as directed on the label, the supplement wouldn't have harmed our intrepid shopper. But the clerk's scientific sounding advice might have. Overdoses of potassium can cause an irregular heart beat and even death.

For most older adults, standard FDAapproved multivitamin-mineral supplements that contain potassium are just fine if taken as directed. It would be virtually impossible for most people to overdose on potassium by eating foods that contain this essential mineral naturally. Some people really do need potassium supplements, as prescribed by a doctor, only, for very specific medical conditions and in very specific, carefully monitored amounts. The point we are making here is that anyone can make scientificsounding claims, but it doesn't necessarily mean that those claims are true or safe. This caution is especially important for people who are on diets with special restrictions — people with kidney disease, congestive heart failure, or diabetes, for example.

Buyer, beware — and check with your doctor before spending your hard-earned money on supplements that promise to restore youthful energy and strength.

Fact: Did you know that your body uses vitamin D to absorb calcium, which makes your bones stronger and helps prevent fractures? Vitamin D is manufactured in the skin following direct exposure to sunlight. The amount of vitamin D produced in the skin varies depending on the time of day, season, latitude, and skin pigmentation.

While many people get enough vitamin D naturally, studies show that vitamin D production decreases in older people and in those who are housebound. These people may need to take vitamin D supplements to ensure a daily intake of between 400 and 800 IU (international units) of vitamin D.

Tips: Major food sources of vitamin D are vitamin D-fortified dairy products, eggs, saltwater fish, dark green vegetables, and liver. Some calcium supplements and most multivitamins contain vitamin D, so it's important to read the labels to find out how much each contains.

Caution: Massive doses of vitamin D may be harmful and are not recommended.

Measuring Progress

When Marty Billowitz throws off his blankets in the morning, he thinks first about his wife Harriet, but seconds later, he is up and moving, pulling on comfortable clothes and lacing up his walking shoes. Where does this 75-year-old grandfather dash off to at 7:00 every morning? Mr. Billowitz goes to the shopping mall — not to get a jump on early-bird bargains, but to join a group of mall-walkers organized by the local hospital. These seniors meet each morning to exercise. Some move at a steady clip through the arteries of the mall, others take a slightly slower pace, but all of the walkers count their laps and keep a daily record of their progress — pushing themselves each day to go a little faster, a little farther.

Mr. Billowitz joined the mall-walkers at his wife's insistence. "Harriet was clear that once I'd retired, no matter what, we were going to walk each morning!" That was nearly 7 years ago. Today Mr. Billowitz says, "The walkers have been a lifeline. They keep me moving on days when all I want to do is sit." You see, Mrs. Billowitz died unexpectedly last year. "It was quite a blow. I always thought I'd be the first to go," he says.

Still, during those years he spent walking miles around mall halls, Mr. Billowitz had done more than just improve his cardiovascular strength...he also had built lasting friendships. It was those friends who brought him back into the walking routine after his wife's death. At first, Mr. Billowitz walked because it was something to do each morning. "But over time, I realized I liked how it felt to be moving. I liked seeing my improvement. Measuring how fast I could walk each morning gave me goals, something to work toward. It also made me feel good to see that I could take care of myself."

Mr. Billowitz believes that the mall-walking habit was a small gift his wife left for him, "I walk and feel stronger every day. That really helps. Some mornings I think of Harriet and silently thank her for insisting that we walk together."

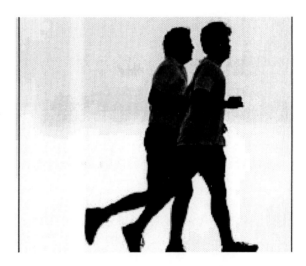

APPENDIX A: TARGET HEART RATE

Target heart rate (THR) is a common way of judging how hard you should exercise during endurance activities. It tells you how fast the average person should try to make his or her heart beat during endurance sessions. It's not always the best way for older adults to decide how hard to exercise, though, because many have long-standing medical conditions or take medications that change their heart rate. We recommend using the Borg scale shown in Section 4 instead. However, some older exercisers who are in basically good health and who like taking a "scientific" approach to their endurance activities may find the THR method useful. Others should check with their doctors first.

For those of you who can use THR, the chart on the next page shows an estimate of how fast you should try to make your heart beat, once you have gradually worked your way up to it. "Gradually" is an important word here.

Going immediately from an inactive lifestyle to exercising at the rate shown in the chart is not advised.

One way to reach your THR gradually is to take your pulse during an endurance-type activity that is already a part of your life (walking, for example). Do it at the pace you normally do it, and record your heart rate. From session to session (or over several sessions), increase how hard you work, so that your pulse rate gradually gets faster, over time.

Eventually, you can try to get your heart rate up to 70 to 85 percent of its maximum ability (the rate shown in the chart). Making it beat faster than this is not advised.

Note: The goal is not for your heart rate to be faster all the time — just when you do your endurance activities. In fact, you should find that, as your heart becomes more efficient from endurance exercise, your resting pulse rate is slower than it was before you took up this healthy habit.

How to Take Your Pulse

To take your pulse, press the tips of your index and middle fingers against the inside of the opposite wrist, just below the mound at the base of your thumb, and count how many pulsations you feel in a 10-second period. Multiplying this number by 6 will give you your heart rate. Don't count your pulse for an entire minute. During the minute that you have stopped exercising to take your pulse, your heart will have slowed down, and you won't get an accurate reading.

Do Not Use the THR Method If...

- You take medications that change your heart rate
- You have a pacemaker for your heart
- You have an irregular heart rhythm called "atrial fibrillation"
- You have any other condition that affects your pulse rate. All of these situations can give you inaccurate readings.

Many older adults take medications in a class called "beta blockers" for high blood pressure or some heart conditions. Your doctor can tell you if your heart or blood-pressure medicine is a beta blocker, or if you have other conditions or medications that will affect your pulse rate during exercise. Some eyedrops used to treat glaucoma also contain beta blockers.

Your heart rate is a reflection of how hard your body is working. Beta blockers tend to keep your heart rate slower, so no matter how hard you push yourself, you might never reach the heart rate you are trying for. You might end up exerting yourself too much, as you try in vain to reach a heart rate that your beta blockers won't allow. Being on beta blockers doesn't mean you can't exercise vigorously; it just means you can't rely on your heart rate or on your pulse rate to judge how hard you are working.

Age	Desired Range for Heart Rate During Endurance Exercise (beats per minute)
40	126- 153
50	119- 145
60	112- 136
70	105- 128
80	98- 119
90	91- 111
100	84- 102

APPENDIX B: EXERCISE PLAN

How Much Exercise Should I Get Each Week?

When you first start out, you might have trouble keeping up with even the minimum amount of exercise we suggest in the chart to the right. Start out with a schedule that your body can tolerate and that you think you really can manage, and build up from there.

Note that the schedules are arranged so that you are never doing strength exercises of the same muscle groups on any two days in a row. If you want to do strength exercises every day, alternate muscle groups. For example, do strength exercises of your upper-body muscles on Monday, Wednesday, and Friday and of your lowerbody muscles on Tuesday, Thursday, and Saturday. Or you can do strength exercises of all of your muscle groups up to every other day.

Begin exercising gradually. Once you have worked your way up to a regular schedule...

...get at least this much exercise each week:

Sunday	Monday	Tuesday	Wednesday	Thursday	Friday	Saturday
	Endurance		Endurance		Endurance	
		Strength/ balance, all muscle groups		Strength/ balance, all muscle groups		
Stretching			Stretching			Stretching

Or ...you can exercise up to this often each week (more than this could cause injuries):

Sunday	Monday	Tuesday	Wednesday	Thursday	Friday	Saturday
Endurance	Endurance	Endurance	Endurance	Endurance	Endurance	Endurance
	Strength/ balance, upper body	Strength/ balance, lower body	Strength/ balance, upper body	Strength/ balance, lower body	Strength/ balance, upper body	Strength/ balance, lower body
Stretching	Stretching	Stretching	Stretching	Stretching	Stretching	Stretching
Anytime, anywhere balance	Anytime, anywhere balance	Anytime, anywhere balance	Anytime, anywhere balance	Anytime, anywhere balance	Anytime, anywhere balance	Anytime, anywhere balance

Appendix C: Activity and Progress Charts

Weekly Schedule

You might want to make copies of this form. Leave this one blank, so you can copy it as needed. Write in the exercises and activities you plan to do. Create a schedule you think you really can manage. You can change your plan as your fitness improves and you are able to do more.

Week of _____

	Endurance	Strength/Balance	Flexibility	Notes
Sunday				
Monday				
Tuesday				
Wednesday				
Thursday				
Friday				
Saturday				

DAILY RECORD

Endurance and Flexibility

You might want to make copies of this form. Leave this one blank, so you can copy it as needed. This form is for keeping track of the activities and exercises you do each day.

Week of _____

	Sunday	Monday	Tuesday	Wednesday	Thursday	Friday	Saturday
Activity:							
Endurance: *List the activity you did and how long you did it.how long?*							
Flexibility. Check the box of each stretching exercise you did:							
Hamstrings							
Alternative Hamstrings							
• Calves							
• Ankles							
• Triceps							
• Wrists							
• Quadriceps							
• Double Hip Rotation							
• Single Hip Rotation							
• Shoulder Rotation							
• Neck Rotation							

Daily Record

Anytime, Anywhere Balance

You might want to make copies of this form. Leave this one blank, so you can copy it as needed. Check the box of each exercise you did.

Week of _____

	Sunday	Monday	Tuesday	Wednesday	Thursday	Friday	Saturday
Anytime, anywhere balance. *Check the box of each exercise you did:*							
Stand on one foot							
Left							
Right							
Stand and sit without using hands							
Walk heel-to-toe							

Strength/Balance

DAILY RECORD

You might want to make copies of this form. Leave this one blank, so you can copy it as needed. This form is for keeping track of the activities and exercises you do each day.

Week of _____

		Sunday	Monday	Tuesday	Wednesday	Thursday	Friday	Saturday
Arm Raise	reps							
	lbs							
Chair Stand	# of stands							
Biceps Curl	Reps							
	lbs							
Plantar Flexion	reps							
	lbs							
Triceps Extension	Reps							
	lbs							
Alternative Dip	# of dips							
Knee Flexion	reps							
	lbs							
Hip Flexion	reps							
	lbs							

		Sunday	Monday	Tuesday	Wednesday	Thursday	Friday	Saturday
Shoulder Flexion	reps							
	lbs							
Knee Extension	reps							
	lbs							
Hip Extension	reps							
	lbs							
Side Leg Raise	reps							
	lbs							

MONTHLY PROGRESS RECORD

Endurance, Lower Body, and Balance

You might want to make copies of this form. Leave this one blank, so you can copy it as needed. Fill out this form on the same day of each month. Compare your scores to see your improvement.

Year _____

	January	February	March	April	May	June	July	August	September	October	November	December
Endurance *Measure how far you are able to walk in 6 minutes. Use the same track and the same unit of measure each time.*												

	January	February	March	April	May	June	July	August	September	October	November	December
Lower–Body Power *Time how fast you can walk up a flight of stairs. Use the same stairs—at least 10 steps—each time.*												
Balance *Time yourself as you stand on one foot, then the other, without support, for as long as you can.*												

Monthly Progress Record

Strength/Balance

You might want to make copies of this form. Leave this one blank, so you can copy it as needed. Fill out this form on the same day of each month. Compare your scores to see your improvement.

Year _____

		January	February	March	April	May	June	July	August	September	October	November	December
Arm Raise	reps												
	lbs												
Chair Stand	# of stands												
Biceps Curl	Reps												
	Lbs												
Plantar Flexion	Reps												
	Lbs												
Triceps Extension	Reps												
	Lbs												
Alternative Dip	# of dips												
Knee Flexion	Reps												
	Lbs												

		January	February	March	April	May	June	July	August	September	October	November	December
Hip Flexion	Reps												
	lbs												
Shoulder Flexion	reps												
	lbs												
Hip Extension	reps												
	lbs												
Side Leg Raise	reps												
	lbs												

APPENDIX D: RESOURCES

Resources

Below are examples of some nonprofit organizations that offer information about exercise and exercise programs for older adults.

American Academy of Orthopedic Surgeons
6300 North River Road
Rosemont, IL 60018-4262
Phone: 1-800-824-BONES
Internet: http://www.aaos.org
Ask for free publications about how to exercise safely.

American College of Sports Medicine
P.O. Box 1440
Indianapolis, IN 46206-1440
Internet: http://www.acsm.org
Send self-addressed, stamped envelope for free brochures on exercise for older adults.

American Diabetes Association
1701 North Beauregard Street
Alexandria, VA 22311
Phone: 1-800-342-2383
Internet: http://www.diabetes.org
Offers free pamphlets about exercise for people of all ages who have diabetes, including "Exercise and Diabetes," "Starting to Exercise," and "20 Steps to Safe Exercise."

American Heart Association
7272 Greenville Avenue
Dallas, TX 75231-4596
Phone: 1-800-242-8721
Internet: http://www.americanheart.org
Offers free pamphlets about exercise for people of all ages.

American Physical Therapy Association
111 North Fairfax Street
Alexandria, VA 22314-1488
Phone: 1-800-999-2782
Internet: http://www.apta.org
Request "For the Young at Heart" (free exercise brochure).

Arthritis Foundation
1330 West Peachtree Street
Atlanta, GA 30309
Phone: 1-800-283-7800
Internet: http://www.arthritis.org
Free pamphlet provides guidelines on how to protect joints during exercise; includes range-of-motion exercises for joint mobility, and others.

Centers for Disease Control and Prevention
1600 Clifton Road
Atlanta, GA 30333
Phone: 1-800-311-3435
Internet: http://www.cdc.gov
Part of US Department of Health and Human Services. Offers physical activity tips and the Surgeon General's Report: "Physical Activity and Health."

Jewish Community Centers
(also appears as Young Men's Hebrew Association or Young Women's Hebrew Association.)
Check phone book for local listing, or call national headquarters at the phone number below.
Phone: (212) 532-4949
Internet: http://www.jcca.org
Most locations offer a variety of exercise and physical activity programs for older adults. All denominations welcome.

National Association of Health and Fitness
201 S. Capitol Avenue, Suite 560
Indianapolis, IN 46225
Phone: (317) 237-5630
Internet: http://www.physicalfitness.org

Sponsors physical-fitness events for older adults. Ask for address and phone number of your State's association.

National Heart, Lung and Blood Institute
NHLBI Information Center
P.O. Box 30105
Bethesda, MD 20824-0105
Phone: (301) 592-8573
Internet: http://www.nhlbi.nih.gov
Part of the National Institutes of Health. Offers free publications, on exercise, diet, and cholesterol.

National Institute of Arthritis and Musculoskeletal and Skin Diseases
National Arthritis and Musculoskeletal and Skin Diseases Information Clearinghouse
1 AMS Circle
Bethesda, MD 20892-3675
Phone: 1-877-22-NIAMS
Internet: http://www.nih.gov/niams/healthinfo/
Part of the National Institutes of Health. Provides free information about exercise and arthritis; large-print copies available on request.

National Institute on Aging
Bldg. 31, Room 5C27
31 Center Drive, MSC 2292
Bethesda, MD 20892-2292
Information Center:
Phone: 1-800-222-2225
TTY: 1-800-222-4225
Internet: http://www.nih.gov/nia
Part of the National Institutes o f Health. Call or write to receive free publications about health and fitness for older adults.

National Osteoporosis Foundation
1232 22nd Street NW.
Washington, DC 20037-1292
Phone: (202) 223-2226
Internet: http://www.nof.org

Call to request free copy of "The Role of Exercise in the Prevention and Treatment of Osteoporosis," "Guidelines for Safe Movement," and "Fall Prevention."

National Senior Games Association
3032 Old Forge Drive
Baton Rouge, LA 70808
Phone: (225) 925-5678
Internet: http://www.nationalseniorgames.org
Conducts summer and winter National Senior Games – The Senior Olympics.

The President's Council on Physical Fitness and Sports
200 Independence Avenue SW.
HHH Bldg., Room 738 H
Washington, DC 20201
Phone: (202) 690-9000
Internet: http://www.fitness.gov
Provides "Pep Up Your Life," a free exercise booklet for older adults, in partnership with AARP.

YMCA and YWCA
Check phone book for local listings.
Services vary from location to location; many offer exercise programs for older adults, including endurance exercises, strength exercises, water exercises, and walking.

CONGRATULATE YOU – OFFICIALLY!

Have you kept up your exercises and activities for more than a month? If so, it's a sign that you are likely to make fitness a lifelong habit. You deserve recognition!

Fill out this form and send it to the address below if you would like to receive an official National Institute on Aging certificate of acknowledgment.

Your Name _____

Your Address

_____

_____

_____

_____

Mail this form to:
NIA Information Center
P.O. Box 8057

Gaithersburg, MD 20898-8057
(Please print clearly)
NIA Information Center
P.O. Box 8057
Gaithersburg, MD 20898-8057

Place Stamp Here

Designed by Levine and Associates, Washington DC

U.S. Department of Health and Human Services
Public Health Service
National Institutes of Health
National Institute on Aging
800-222-2225
http://www.nih.gov/nia
NIH Publication No. 01-4258

ACKNOWLEDGMENTS

The National Institute on Aging, part of the National Institutes of Health, brought together some of the nation's best-informed experts on the topic of exercise for older adults to discuss the writing of this book.
They include:

Panel co-chairpersons: Chhanda Dutta, Ph.D.,
and **Marcia Ory, Ph.D.**; Health Scientist
Administrators; National Institute on Aging,
National Institutes of Health

David Buchner, M.D., M.P.H.;
Professor, Department of Health Services,
University of Washington

Marie Elaine Cress, Ph.D.; Associate Professor,
Department of Exercise Science and Gerontology
Center, University of Georgia

William Evans, Ph.D.; Director of Nutrition,
Metabolism, and Exercise Laboratory at Donald W.
Reynolds Department of Geriatrics, University of
Arkansas for Medical Sciences

Maria Fiatarone Singh, M.D.; Associate
Professor, School of Nutrition and Science Policy,
Tufts University

Alan Jette, Ph.D.; Dean, Sargent College of Health
and Rehabilitation Sciences, Boston University

Thomas R. Prohaska, Ph.D.; Director, Center for
Research on Health and Aging, University of
Illinois at Chicago

Anita Stewart, Ph.D.; Professor in Residence,
Institute for Health and Aging, University of
California San Francisco

We also extend special thanks to Steven N. Blair, P.E.D., Director of
Research at the Cooper Institute for Aerobics Research; and to Roger
Fielding, Ph.D., Assistant Professor of Health Sciences and Brookdale
National Fellow at the Sargent College of Health and Rehabilitation
Sciences, Boston University, for their contributions.

Each of these experts is a major force in research devoted to improving
the health and independence of older adults through exercise. We are
grateful to them and to other leaders in the field whose work is reflected in
these pages for sharing their expertise.

We are also grateful to Jerome L. Fleg, M.D., and Edward G. Lakatta,
M.D., of the Gerontology Research Center; the American College of Sports
Medicine; the American Heart Association; the American Physical Therapy

Association; the National Center for Medical Rehabilitation and Research; the National Heart, Lung and Blood Institute; the National Institute of Arthritis and Musculoskeletal and Skin Diseases; the National Institute of Child Health and Human Development; the Office of Disease Prevention of the National Institutes of Health; the National Aeronautics and Space Administration; and the Public Health Service Office on Women's Health.

In: Guide to Physical Fitness and Exercise ISBN 1-59454-737-8
Editor: Pamela B. Carter, pp. 83-92 © 2006 Nova Science Publishers, Inc.

Chapter 2

EXERCISE AND WEIGHT CONTROL[*]

President's Council on Physical Fitness and Sports

Just about everybody seems to be interested in weight control. Some of us weigh just the right amount, others need to gain a few pounds. Most of us "battle the bulge" at some time in our life. Whatever our goals, we should understand and take advantage of the important role of exercise in keeping our weight under control.

Carrying around too much body fat is a major nuisance. Yet excess body fat is common in modern-day living. Few of today's occupations require vigorous physical activity, and much of our leisure time is spent in sedentary pursuits. Recent estimates indicate that 34 million adults are considered obese (20 percent above desirable weight). Also, there has been an increase in body fat levels in children and youth over the past 20 years. After infancy and early childhood, the earlier the onset of obesity, the greater the likelihood of remaining obese.

Excess body fat has been linked to such health problems as coronary heart disease, high blood pressure, osteoporosis, diabetes, arthritis and certain forms of cancer. Some evidence now exists showing that obesity has a negative effect on both health and longevity.

Exercise is associated with the loss of body fat in both obese and normal weight persons. A regular program of exercise is an important component of any plan to help individuals lose, gain or maintain their weight.

---

[*] Extracted from http://www.fitness.gov/exerciseweight.htm

OVERWEIGHT OR OVERFAT?

Overweight and overfat do not always mean the same thing. Some people are quite muscular and weigh more than the average for their age and height. However, their body composition, the amount of fat versus lean body mass (muscle, bone, organs and tissue), is within a desirable range. This is true for many athletes. Others weigh an average amount yet carry around too much fat. In our society, however, overweight often implies overfat because excess weight is commonly distributed as excess fat. The addition of exercise to a weight control program helps control both body weight and body fat levels. A certain amount of body fat is necessary for everyone. Experts say that percent body fat for women should be about 20 percent, 15 percent for men. Women with more than 30 percent fat and men with more than 25 percent fat are considered obese. How much of your weight is fat can be assessed by a variety of methods including underwater (hydrostatic) weighing, skinfold thickness measurements and circumference measurements. Each requires a specially trained person to administer the test and perform the correct calculations. From the numbers obtained, a body fat percentage is determined. Assessing body composition has an advantage over the standard height-weight tables because it can help distinguish between "overweight" and "overfat." An easy self-test you can do is to pinch the thickness of the fat folds at your waist and abdomen. If you can pinch an inch or more of fat (make sure no muscle is included) chances are you have too much body fat. People who exercise appropriately increase lean body mass while decreasing their overall fat level. Depending on the amount of fat loss, this can result in a loss of inches *without* a loss of weight, since muscle weighs more than fat. However, with the proper combination of diet and exercise, both body fat and overall weight can be reduced.

ENERGY BALANCE: A WEIGHTY CONCEPT

Losing weight, gaining weight or maintaining your weight depends on the amount of calories you take in and use up during the day, otherwise referred to as energy balance. Learning how to balance energy intake (calories in food) with energy output (calories expended through physical activity) will help you achieve your desired weight. Although the underlying causes and the treatments of obesity are complex, the concept of energy balance is relatively simple. If you eat more calories than your body needs to perform your day's activities, the extra calories are stored as fat. If you do not take in enough calories to meet your body's energy needs, your body will go to the stored fat to make up the difference (Exercise helps ensure that stored fat, rather than muscle tissue, is used to meet your energy needs.) If you eat just about the same amount of calories to meet your body's energy needs, your weight will stay the same. On the average, a person consumes between 800,000 and 900,000 calories each year! An active person needs more calories than a sedentary person, as physically active people require energy above and beyond the day's basic needs. All too often, people who want to lose weight concentrate on counting calorie intake while neglecting calorie output. The most powerful formula is the combination of dietary modification with exercise. By increasing your daily physical activity and decreasing your caloric input you can lose excess weight in the most efficient and healthful way.

Counting Calories

Each pound of fat your body stores represents 3,500 calories of unused energy. In order to lose one pound, you would have to create a calorie deficit of 3,500 calories by either taking in 3,500 less calories over a period of time than you need or doing 3,500 calories worth of exercise. It is recommended that no more than two pounds (7,000 calories) be lost per week for lasting weight loss.

Adding 15 minutes of moderate exercise, say walking one mile, to your daily schedule will use up 100 extra calories per day. (Your body uses approximately 100 calories of energy to walk one mile, depending on your body weight.) Maintaining this schedule would result in an extra 700 calories per week used up, or a loss of about 10 pounds in one year, assuming your food intake stays the same. To look at energy balance another way, just one extra slice of bread or one extra soft drink a day – or any other food that contains approximately 100 calories – can add up to ten extra pounds in a year if the amount of physical activity you do does not increase. If you already have a lean figure and want to keep it you should exercise regularly and eat a balanced diet that provides enough calories to make up for the energy you expend. If you wish to gain weight you should exercise regularly and increase the number of calories you consume until you reach your desired weight. Exercise will help ensure that the weight you gain will be lean muscle mass, not extra fat.

THE DIET CONNECTION

A balanced diet should be part of any weight control plan. A diet high in complex carbohydrates and moderate in protein and fat will complement an exercise program. It should include enough calories to satisfy your daily nutrient requirements and include the proper number of servings per day from the "basic four food groups": vegetables and fruits (4 servings), breads and cereals (4 servings), milk and milk products (2 - 4 depending on age) and meats and fish (2). Experts recommend that your daily intake not fall below 1200 calories unless you are under a doctor's supervision. Also, weekly weight loss should not exceed two pounds. Remarkable claims have been made for a variety of "crash" diets and diet pills. And some of these very restricted diets do result in noticeable weight loss in a short time. Much of this loss is water and such a loss is quickly regained when normal food and liquid intake is resumed. These diet plans are often expensive and may be dangerous. Moreover, they do not emphasize lifestyle changes that will help you maintain your desired weight. Dieting alone will result in a loss of valuable body tissue such as muscle mass in addition to a loss in fat.

HOW MANY CALORIES

The estimates for number of calories (energy) used during a physical activity are based on experiments that measure the amount of oxygen consumed during a specific bout of exercise for a certain body weight. The energy costs of activities that require you to move your own body weight, such as walking or jogging, are greater for heavier people since they have more weight to move. For example, a person weighing 150 pounds would use more calories jogging one mile than a person jogging alongside who weighs 115 pounds. Always check to see what body weight is referred to in caloric expenditure charts you use.

Energy Expenditure Chart

	Energy Costs
A. Sedentary Activities	**Cals/Hour***
Lying down or sleeping	90
Sitting quietly	84
Sitting and writing, card playing, etc .	114
B. Moderate Activities	**(150-350)**
Bicycling (5 mph)	174
Canoeing (2.5 mph)	174
Dancing (Ballroom)	210
Golf (2-some, carrying clubs)	324
Horseback riding (sitting to trot)	246
Light housework, cleaning, etc.	246
Swimming (crawl, 20 yards/min)	288
Tennis (recreational doubles)	312
Volleyball (recreational)	264
Walking (2 mph)	198
C. Vigorous Activities	**More than 350**
Aerobic Dancing	546
Basketball (recreational)	450
Bicycling (13 mph)	612
Circuit weight training	756
Football (touch, vigorous)	498
Ice Skating (9 mph)	384
Racquetball	588
Roller Skating (9 mph)	384
Jogging (10 minute mile, 6 mph)	654
Scrubbing Floors	440
Swimming (crawl, 45 yards/min)	522
Tennis (recreational singles)	450
X-country Skiing (5 mph)	690

*Hourly estimates based on values calculated for calories burned per minute for a 150 pound (68 kg) person.

*(Sources: "William D. McArdle, Frank I. Katch, Victor L. Katch, "Exercise Physiology: Energy, Nutrition and Human Performance" (2nd edition), Lea and Febiger, Philadelphia, 1986; Melvin H. Williams, "Nutrition for Fitness and Sport," William C. Brown Company Publishers, Dubuque, 1983.)

EXERCISE AND MODERN LIVING

One thing is certain. Most people do not get enough exercise in their ordinary routines. All of the advances of modern technology – from electric can openers to power steering – have made life easier, more comfortable and much less physically demanding. Yet our bodies need activity, especially if they are carrying around too much fat. Satisfying this need requires a definite plan, and a commitment. There are two main ways to increase the number of calories you expend:

1. Start a regular exercise program if you do not have one already.
2. Increase the amount of physical activity in your daily routine.

The best way to control your weight is a combination of the above. The sum total of calories used over time will help regulate your weight as well as keep you physically fit.

Active Lifestyles

Before looking at what kind of regular exercise program is best, let's look at how you can increase the amount of physical activity in your daily routine to supplement your exercise program.

- Recreational pursuits such as gardening on weekends, bowling in the office league, family outings, an evening of social dancing, and many other activities provide added exercise. They are fun and can be considered an extra bonus in your weight control campaign.
- Add more "action" to your day. Walk to the neighborhood grocery store instead of using the car. Park several blocks from the office and walk the rest of the way. Walk up the stairs instead of using the elevator; start with one flight of steps and gradually increase.
- Change your attitude toward movement. Instead of considering an extra little walk or trip to the files an annoyance, look upon it as an added fitness boost. Look for opportunities to use your body. Bend, stretch, reach, move, lift and carry. Time-saving devices and gadgets eliminate drudgery and are a bonus to mankind, but when they substitute too often for physical activity they can demand a high cost in health, vigor and fitness.

These little bits of action are cumulative in their effects. Alone, each does not burn a huge amount of calories. But when added together they can result in a sizable amount of energy used over the course of the day. And they will help improve your muscle tone and flexibility at the same time.

WHAT KIND OF EXERCISE?

Although any kind of physical movement requires energy (calories), the type of exercise that uses the most energy is aerobic exercise. The term "aerobic" is derived from the Greek word meaning "with oxygen." Jogging, brisk walking, swimming, biking, cross-country skiing and aerobic dancing are some popular forms of aerobic exercise.

Aerobic exercises use the body's large muscle groups in continuous, rhythmic, sustained movement and require oxygen for the production of energy. When oxygen is combined with food (which can come from stored fat) energy is produced to power the body's musculature. The longer you move aerobically, the more energy needed and the more calories used. Regular aerobic exercise will improve your cardiorespiratory endurance, the ability of your heart, lungs, blood vessels and associated tissues to use oxygen to produce energy needed for activity. You'll build a healthier body while getting rid of excess body fat. In addition to the aerobic exercise, supplement your program with muscle strengthening and stretching exercises. The stronger your muscles, the longer you will be able to keep going during aerobic activity, and the less chance of injury.

How Much? How Often?

Experts recommend that you do some form of aerobic exercise at least three times a week for a minimum of 20 continuous minutes. Of course, if that is too much, start with a shorter time span and gradually build up to the minimum. Then gradually progress until you are able to work aerobically for 20-40 minutes. If you need to lose a large amount of weight, you may want to do your aerobic workout five times a week. It is important to exercise at an intensity vigorous enough to cause your heart rate and breathing to increase. How hard you should exercise depends to a certain degree on your age, and is determined by measuring your heart rate in beats per minute. The heart rate you should maintain is called your target heart rate, and there are several ways you can arrive at this figure. The simplest is to subtract your age from 220 and then calculate 60 to 80 percent of that figure. Beginners should maintain the 60 percent level, more advanced can work up to the 80 percent level. This is just a guide however, and people with any medical limitations should discuss this formula with their physician. You can do different types of aerobic activities, say walking one day, riding a bike the next. Make sure you choose an activity that can be done regularly, and is enjoyable for you. The important thing to remember is not to skip too many days between workouts or fitness benefits will be lost. If you must lose a few days, gradually work back into your routine.

THE BENEFITS OF EXERCISE IN A WEIGHT CONTROL PROGRAM

The benefits of exercise are many, from producing physically fit bodies to providing an outlet for fun and socialization. When added to a weight control program these benefits take on increased significance. We already have noted that proper exercise can help control weight by burning excess body fat. It also has two other body-trimming advantages 1) exercise builds muscle tissue and muscle uses calories up at a faster rate than body fat; and 2) exercise helps reduce inches and a firm, lean body looks slimmer even if your weight remains the same. Remember, fat does not "turn into" muscle, as is often believed. Fat and muscle are two entirely different substances and one cannot become the other. However, muscle does use calories at a faster rate than fat which directly affects your body's metabolic rate or energy requirement. Your basal metabolic rate (BMR) is the amount of energy required to sustain the body's functions at rest and it depends on your age, sex, body size, genes and body composition. People with high levels of muscle tend to have higher BMRs and use more calories in the resting stage. Some studies have even shown that your metabolic rate stays elevated for some time after vigorous exercise, causing you to use even more calories throughout your day. Additional benefits may be seen in how exercise affects appetite. A lean person in good shape may eat more following increased activity, but the regular exercise will burn up the extra calories consumed. On the other hand, vigorous exercise has been reported to suppress appetite. And, physical activity can be used as a positive substitute for between meal snacking.

Better Mental Health

The psychological benefits of exercise are equally important to the weight conscious person. Exercise decreases stress and relieves tensions that might otherwise lead to overeating. Exercise builds physical fitness which in turn builds self-confidence, enhanced self-image, and a positive outlook. When you start to feel good about yourself, you are more likely to want to make other positive changes in your lifestyle that will help keep your weight under control. In addition, exercise can be fun, provide recreation and offer opportunities for companionship. The exhilaration and emotional release of participating in sports or other activities are a boost to mental and physical health. Pent-up anxieties and frustrations seem to disappear when you're concentrating on returning a serve, sinking a putt or going that extra mile.

TIPS TO GET YOU STARTED

Hopefully, you are now convinced that in order to successfully manage your weight you must include exercise in your daily routine. Here are some tips to get you started:

1. Check with your doctor first. Since you are carrying around some extra "baggage," it is wise to get your doctor's "OK" before embarking on an exercise program.
2. Choose activities that you think you'll enjoy. Most people will stick to their exercise program if they are having fun, even though they are working hard.
3. Set aside a regular exercise time. Whether this means joining an exercise class or getting up a little earlier every day, make time for this addition to your routine and don't let anything get in your way. Planning ahead will help you get around interruptions in your workout schedule, such as bad weather and vacations.
4. Set short term goals. Don't expect to lose 20 pounds in two weeks. It has taken awhile for you to gain the weight, it will take time to lose it. Keep a record of your progress and tell your friends and family about your achievements.
5. Vary your exercise program. Change exercises or invite friends to join you to make your workout more enjoyable. There is no "best" exercise – just the one that works best for you. It won't be easy, especially at the start. But as you begin to feel better, look better

and enjoy a new zest for life, you will be rewarded many times over for your efforts.

TIPS TO KEEP YOU GOING

1. Adopt a specific plan and write it down.
2. Keep setting realistic goals as you go along, and remind yourself of them often.
3. Keep a log to record your progress and make sure to keep it up-to-date.
4. Include weight and/or percent body fat measures in your log. Extra pounds can easily creep back.
5. Upgrade your fitness program as you progress.
6. Enlist the support and company of your family and friends.
7. Update others on your successes.
8. Avoid injuries by pacing yourself and including a warmup and cool down period as part of every workout.
9. Reward yourself periodically for a job well done!

INDEX

Guide to Physical Fitness and Exercise

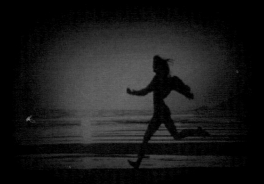

Pamela B. Carter
Editor

ISBN 1-59454-737-8